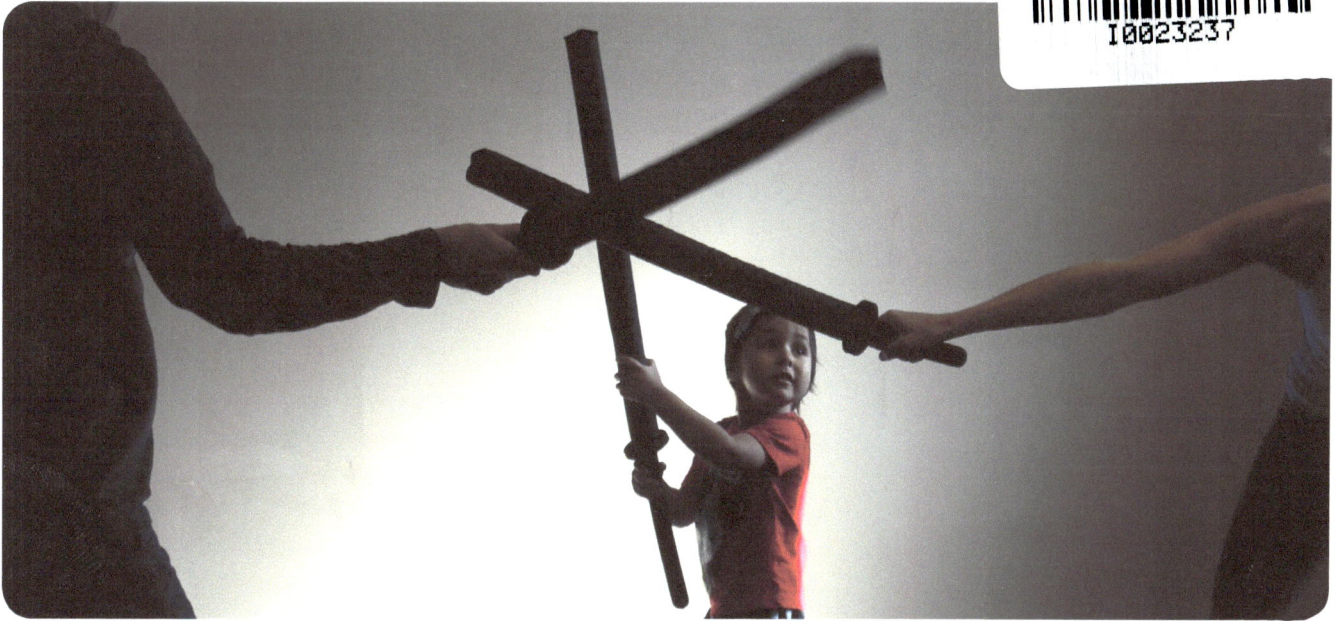

Photo by Andie Baker

This book is dedicated to my nephew, Judah, whose curiosity on a quiet Sunday morning sparked the inspiration for this book.

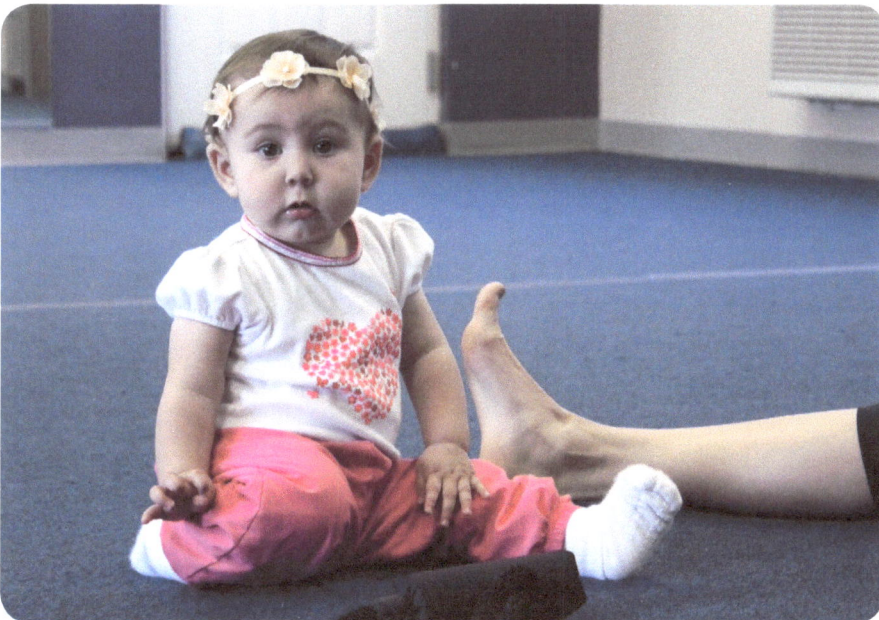

This book is also dedicated to my niece, Posey Poo.

Even though she wasn't born yet when the idea of this book started, little sisters rule and deserve to have books dedicated to them.

Photo by Andie Baker

Love you both, Judah and Posey.
Can't wait to continue kung fu and yoga camp when you're older!

Special thank you...

Grandmaster Sin Thé

For sharing your knowledge and teaching us amazing things, including these exercises. We are all truly grateful for what you've shared with us.

Husband, Master Joe Harmon

For loving me and supporting me through everything. I could write a book for how much appreciation I have for you. Can't wait to get old and still conquer mountains with you.

Master Dennis & Master Jerome Cook

For being my first martial arts teachers and teaching me the details of these exercises as you learned from Grandmaster Sin. I sincerely appreciate all the help you've given me over the years and the help you've given me to compile this book.

Amber Gean

For being one of my absolute favorite yoga teachers, and whose teachings helped inspire many of the variations in this book.

Sunday ICC Class

For showing up week after week to "Katy's House of Pain." And for putting up with my evil experiments on how to make ICC class even harder.

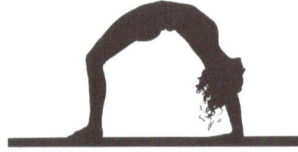

Ordering Information:
Available from Amazon.com, CreateSpace.com, and other retail outlets.

Printed in the USA

CreateSpace, An Amazon.com Company
Charleston SC
www.createspace.com

ISBN-10:0991435508
ISBN-13:978-0-9914355-0-0

Photographer: Rick Lohre
Editor: Robyn Holleran
Layout Designer: Ryan Noga

Medical Disclaimer

As with any new physical activity, please consult your doctor before attempting any of the exercises
showcased in this book. Attempt the exercises at your own risk. Total Body Arts LLC, Katy Moeggenberg,
or any affiliate of Shaolin-Do under Grandmaster Sin Thé shall not be held responsible for any injury or
death resulting in attempting the exercises contained in this book.

I Chin Ching

49 Exercises to Build Strength,

Increase Flexibility, &

Improve Balance

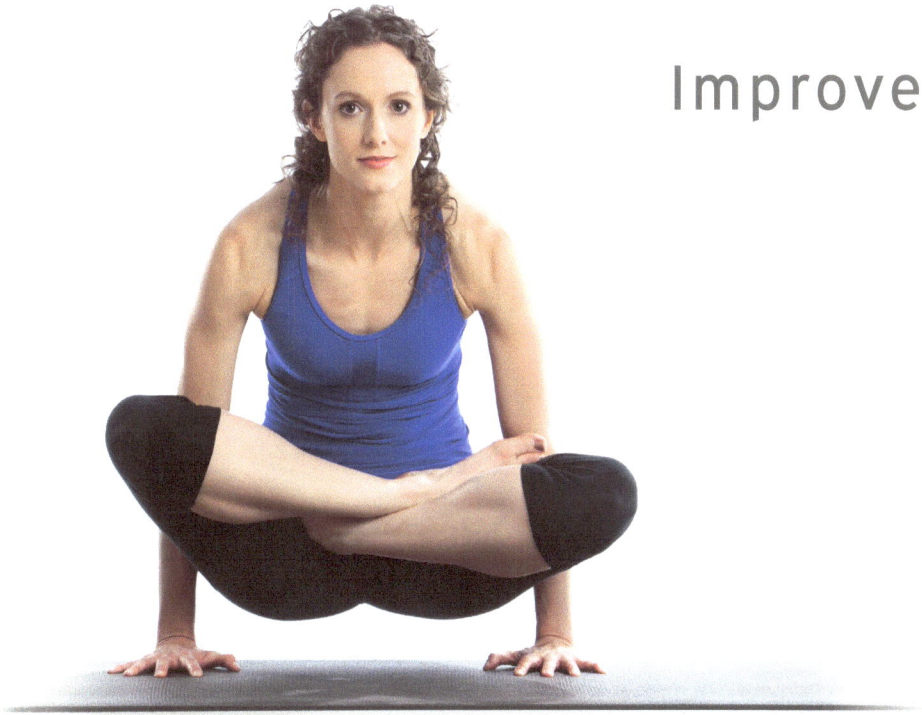

Katy Moeggenberg

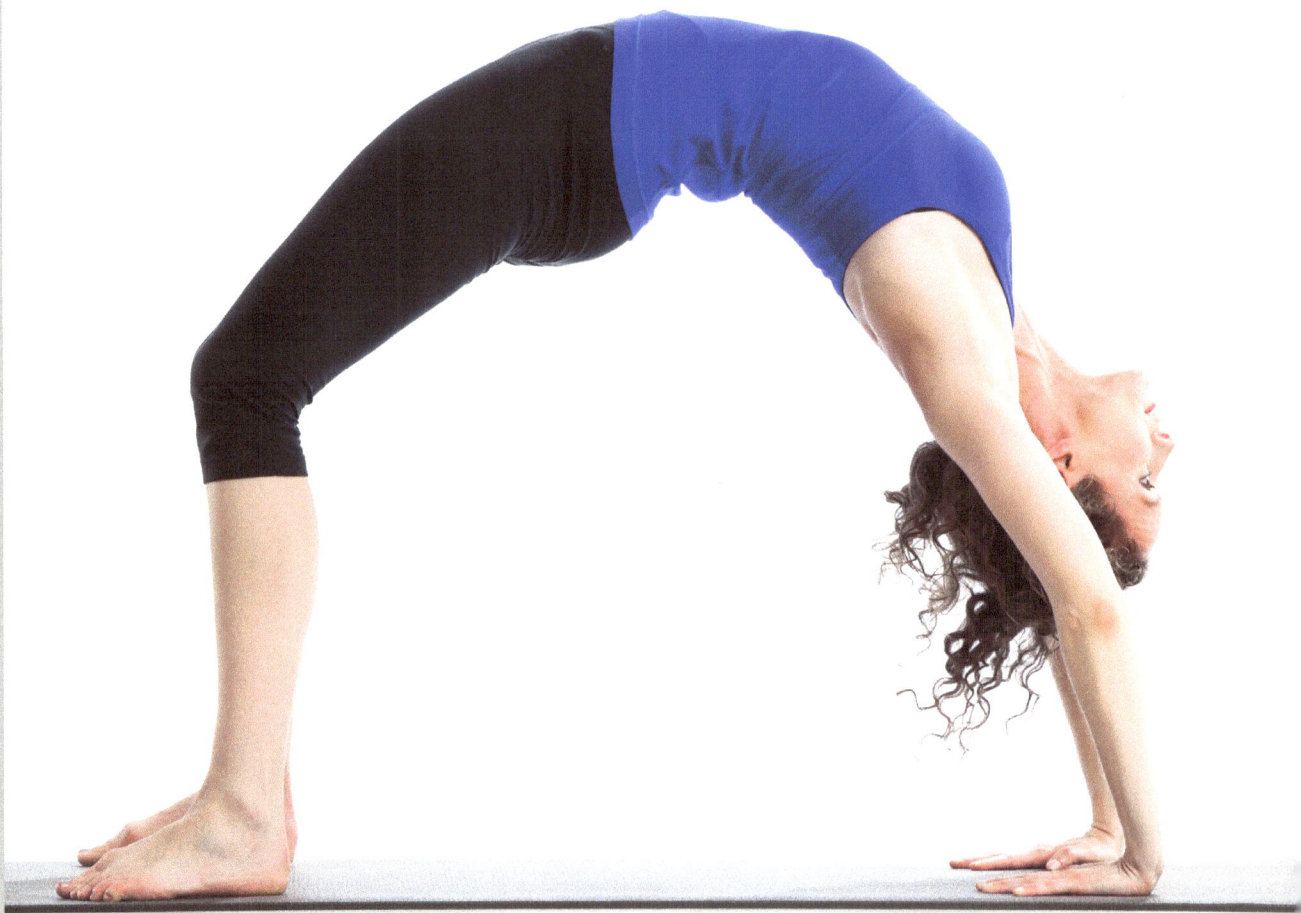

Thank you for purchasing this book! I sincerely appreciate your support and I hope practicing I Chin Ching does as much for you as it has done for me.
`

The objectives of this book are threefold:

1. Share the knowledge as it was taught to me, as I've received significant physical benefits from practicing these exercises

2. Provide a visual manual on how to do the exercises with proper technique

3. Provide realistic variations to help you build strength and flexibility so you can eventually achieve some of the tougher exercises

For perspective, it has taken me over 10 years to be able to do all 49 exercises and a few of the really tough exercises I can only do for a few moments (fortunately I have a quick photographer). The variations will come in handy.

Please note that the variations were made up entirely by me, based on my dance and yoga background and my experience teaching I Chin Ching since the early 2000s. These variations do not represent how Shaolin monks may have practiced the exercises throughout history.

Meaning & History

I Chin Ching or Yijin jing stands for "muscle/tendon change classic" or the "change of tendon and muscle." The idea is that by tensing your muscles through static holds/stretches and dynamic motions , you can build stronger, more flexible muscles and tendons, while achieving better balance and coordination. That's a lot of promise for just 49 exercises!

There are many legends on I Chin Ching and how it came to be. Some of the legends are vague and some are contradictory so I will share a brief history based on what I was taught and will focus the majority of the book on the exercises themselves.

The legend I was taught indicates that Bodhidharma, a Buddhist monk from India, traveled the Himalayan mountains to bring Buddhism to China. As he encountered the Shaolin monasteries, Bodhidharma found the monks to be very weak and unable to sustain long meditations. Therefore he taught the monks several exercises to change their physical bodies and build stronger, more flexible muscles which would result in even stronger minds. These exercises became known as the I Chin Ching exercises.

Many of the exercises are similar to or are exact replicas of yoga postures, perhaps as an influence from Bodhidharma's Indian roots.

In addition to multiple legends about the history, there are multiple accounts about how many exercises were in the original set. Some sources indicate there were 12, 18, 24, or even 30. I was taught 49 and therefore this book will focus on those particular 49. One could hypothesize that more exercises were added over time to work various parts of the body. For example, I have made up my own variations and partner exercises using the same breathing and tension techniques in an attempt to train and change my muscles and tendons in different ways. Those exercises may be featured in future books.

Additional sources on the history can be found online if you are interested in studying more.

Basic Breathing Technique

The majority of the I Chin Ching exercises have a very specific breathing pattern: inhale through your nose, then exhale forcefully through your teeth to make a loud hissing sound.

Focus on "even in/even out" breathing. Said differently, inhale for the same number of counts that you exhale. There isn't a magic number of counts as people may count at different speeds or hold the exercises for different amounts of time. Starting out, target a 4 count inhalation and a 4 count exhalation and adjust as needed.

Be mindful of the "even in/even out" concept. It's very easy to form a bad habit and take short inhalations with long exhalations, which can result in dizziness or even fainting.

There are a few I Chin Ching exercises that have breath holds and normal exhalations (no hissing sound) throughout the course of the exercise. I will note the breath change on those particular exercises (#8, #9, #10, #11, #12).

Exercise Classifications

The I Chin Ching exercises can be classified into 5 groups:

1 Static Tension – holding a static position and tensing muscles without moving or changing the muscle length

2 Moving Tension – moving through an exercise while tensing the focused muscles throughout the entire motion and likely the muscle length changes throughout the exercise

3 Moving without Tension – moving through an exercise without tensing any muscles throughout the entire motion

4 Stretching Tension – performing a stretch while pushing farther into the stretch and tensing the stretched muscles

5 Stretching without Tension – performing a stretch while pushing farther into the stretch without tensing the stretched muscles

Many of the I Chin Ching exercises could be classified as isometric or isotonic; however, for simplicity, you can refer to them in the above mentioned classifications.

The first several exercises may seem simple; however they offer critical foundation to safely and successfully achieving some of the later, tougher exercises. For example:

• Exercises #1 and #2 help you develop the needed wrist and forearm strength to hold exercises like #43 and #49

• Exercises #16 and #17 help you develop the upper back and hamstring strength to hold #25

The legend indicates that the monks eventually trained to do these 49 exercises for 49 repetitions daily. Depending on the cadence of your breath, this could take anywhere from 6-8 hours!   Legend also indicates that certain monks did 7 exercises a day for 49 repetitions, so they could get to every exercise each week.

In my weekly hour class, we target 7-14 repetitions for 25-30 exercises. For your own practice, start with a small number of repetitions and gradually increase over time as you build more strength and flexibility.

The Exercises

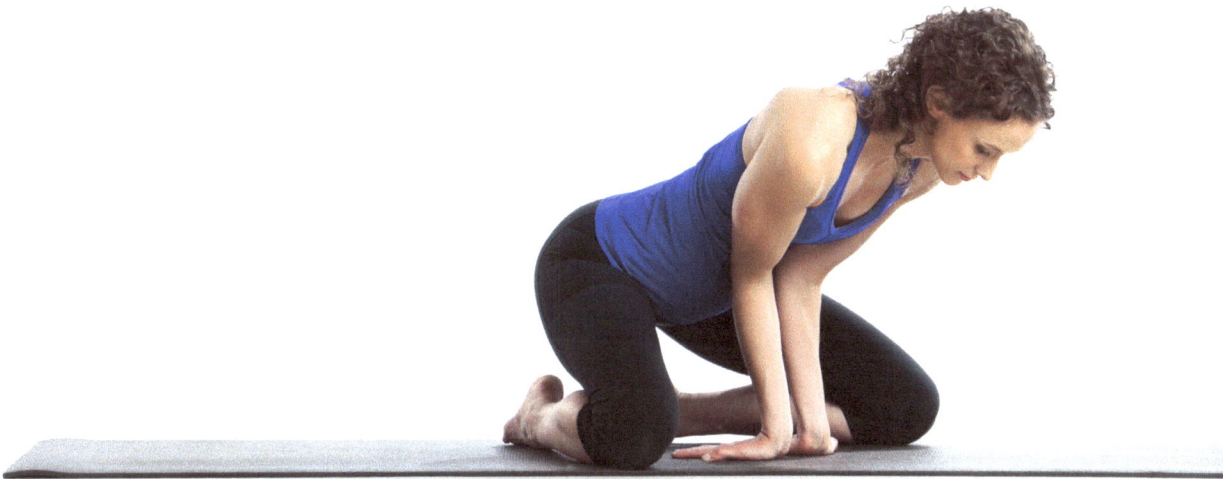

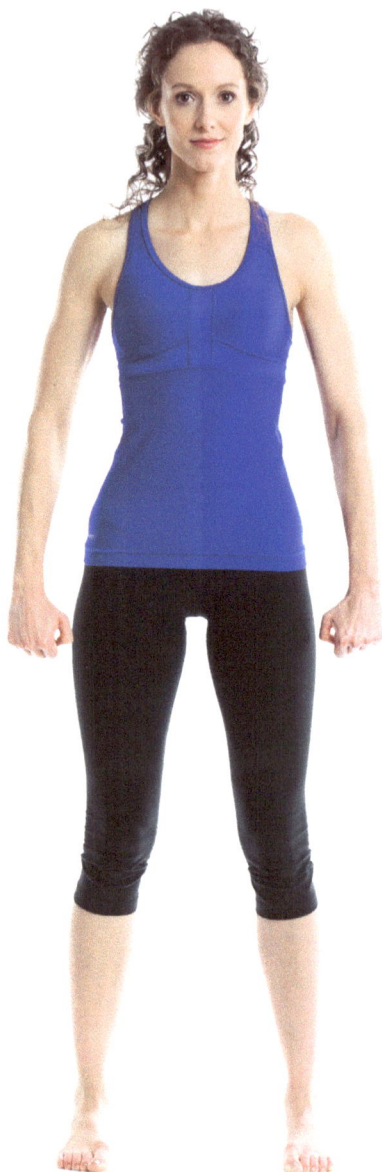

A

Stand straight with your feet shoulder width apart, knees slightly bent, and arms by your sides.

Clench your hands into fists.
Inhale.

B

Exhale as you bring your knuckles up and tense the front of your forearms.

Hold position **B** on each inhalation and tense harder while bringing your knuckles closer to your forearms on each exhalation.

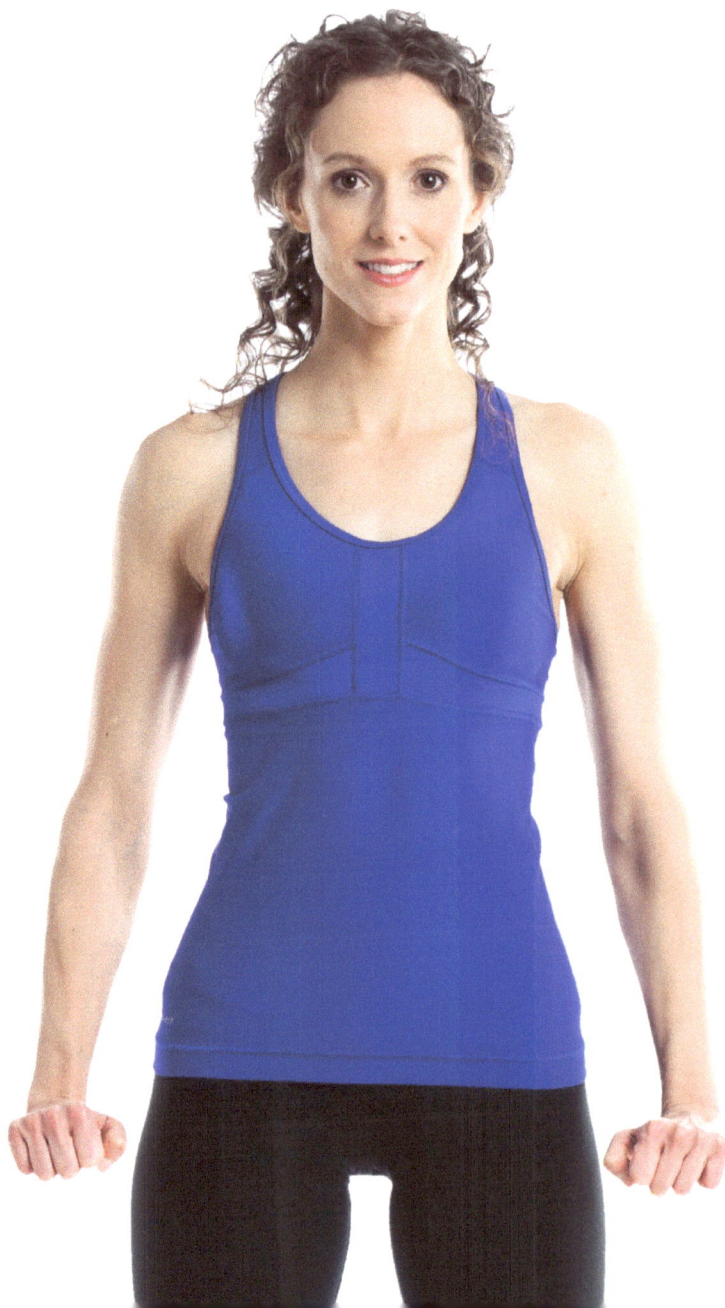

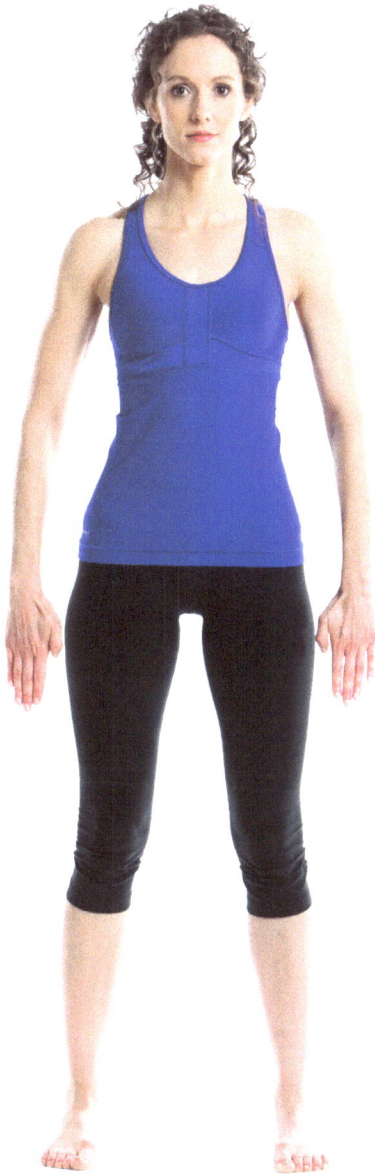

A

Stand straight with your feet shoulder width apart, knees slightly bent, and arms by your sides.

Flatten your hands with your palms facing behind you.
Inhale.

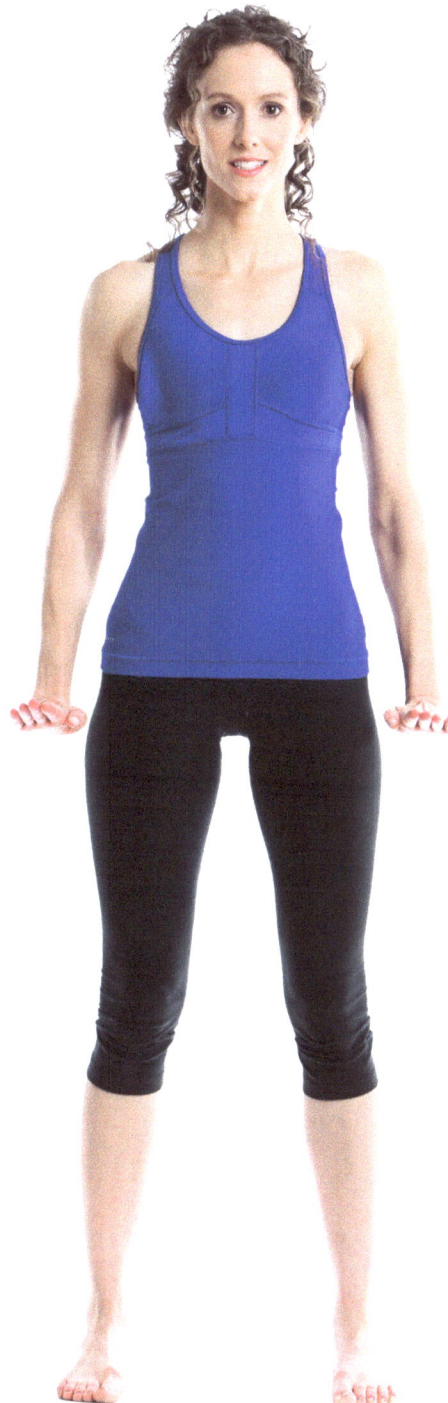

B

Exhale as you bring your fingertips up, including your thumbs, so that your palms face the floor.

Tense the front of your forearms.

Hold position **B** on each inhalation and tense harder while bringing your fingertips closer to the forearm on each exhalation.

3

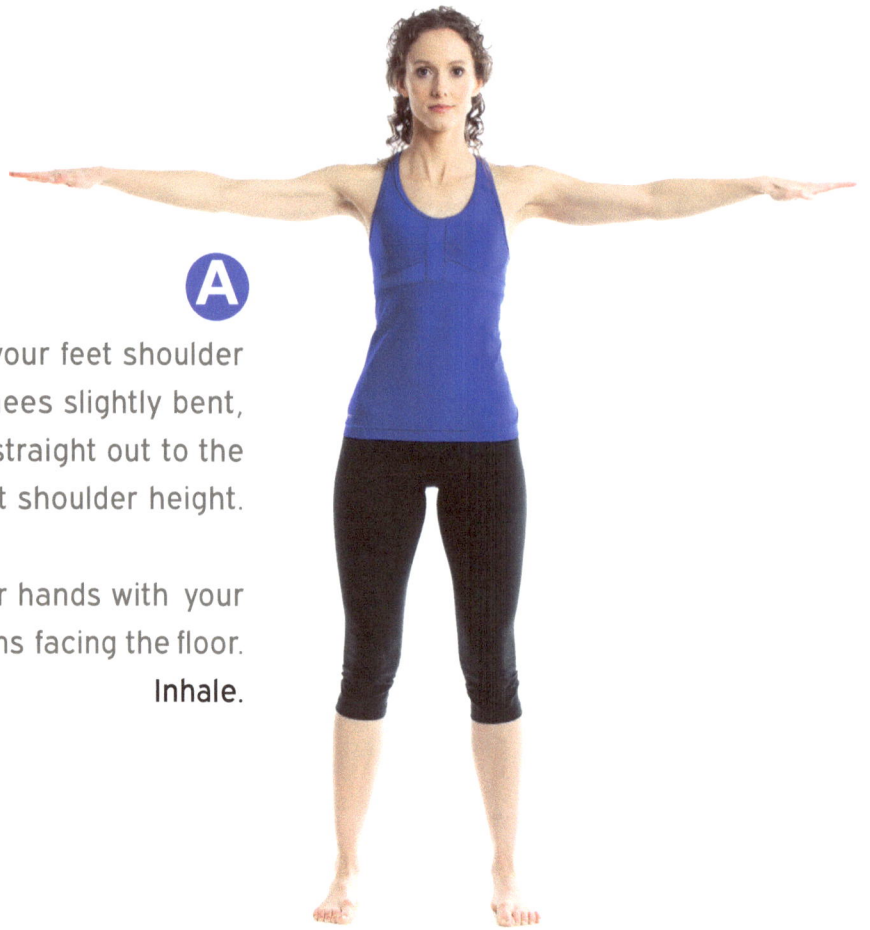

A

Stand straight with your feet shoulder width apart, knees slightly bent, and arms straight out to the side at shoulder height.

Flatten your hands with your palms facing the floor. **Inhale.**

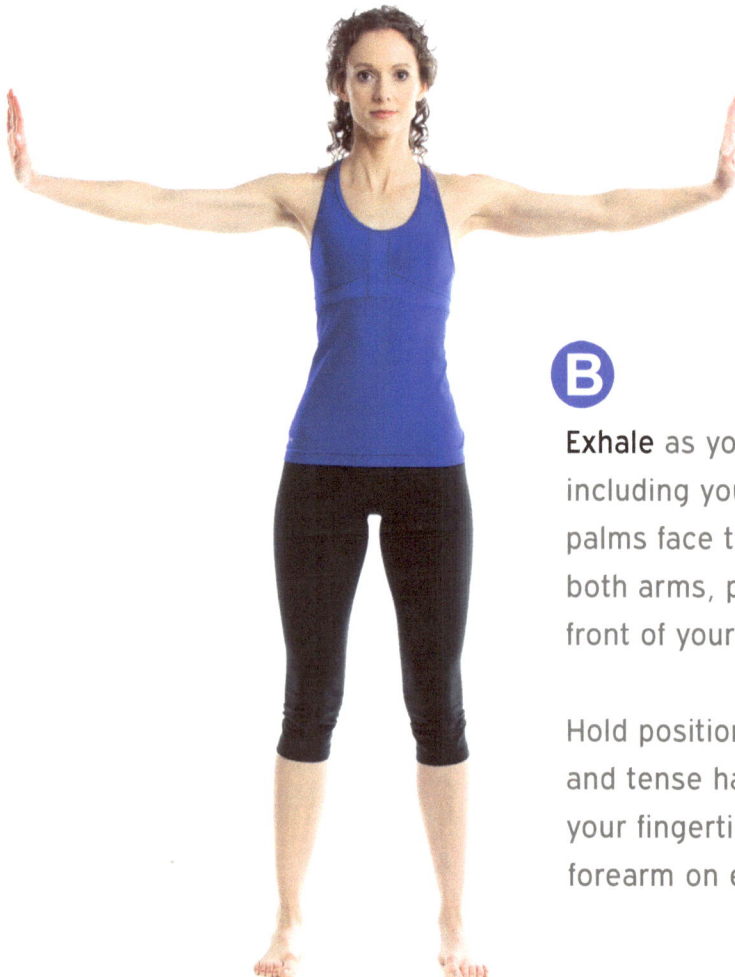

B

Exhale as you bring your fingertips up, including your thumbs, so that your palms face the side and tense both arms, particularly the front of your forearms.

Hold position **B** on each inhalation and tense harder while bringing your fingertips closer to your forearm on each exhalation.

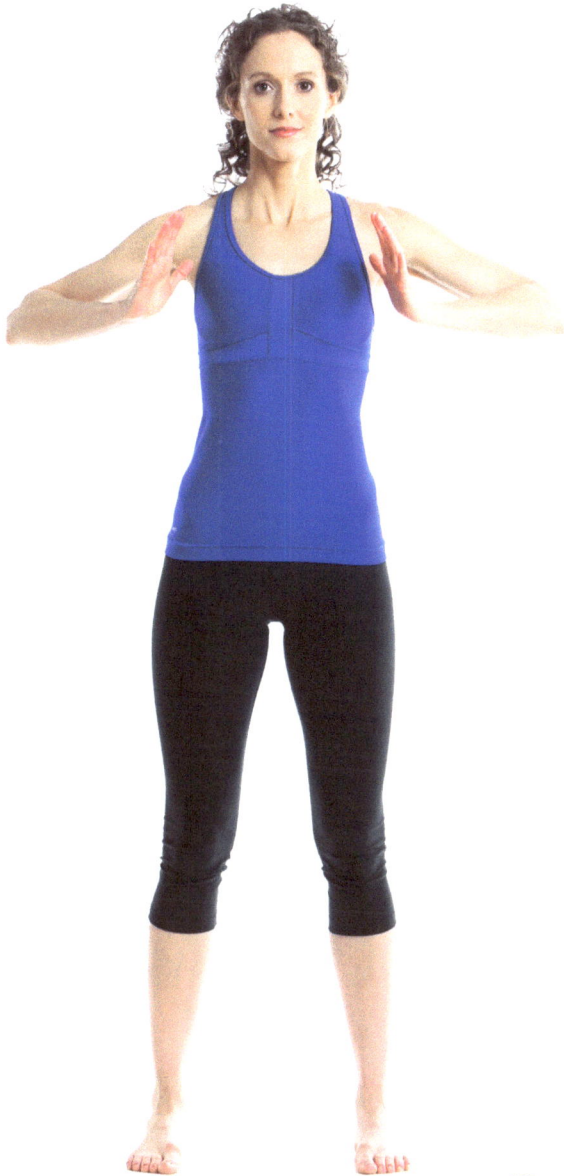

A

Stand straight with your feet shoulder width apart, knees slightly bent, and your hands in at your shoulders. **Inhale**.

B

Exhale as you press your hands together as if you are pushing opposing magnets together. Tense your chest and biceps.

Pull your hands apart, back to position **A**, on each inhalation with no tension.

Press your hands together, back to position **B**, and tense harder on each exhalation.

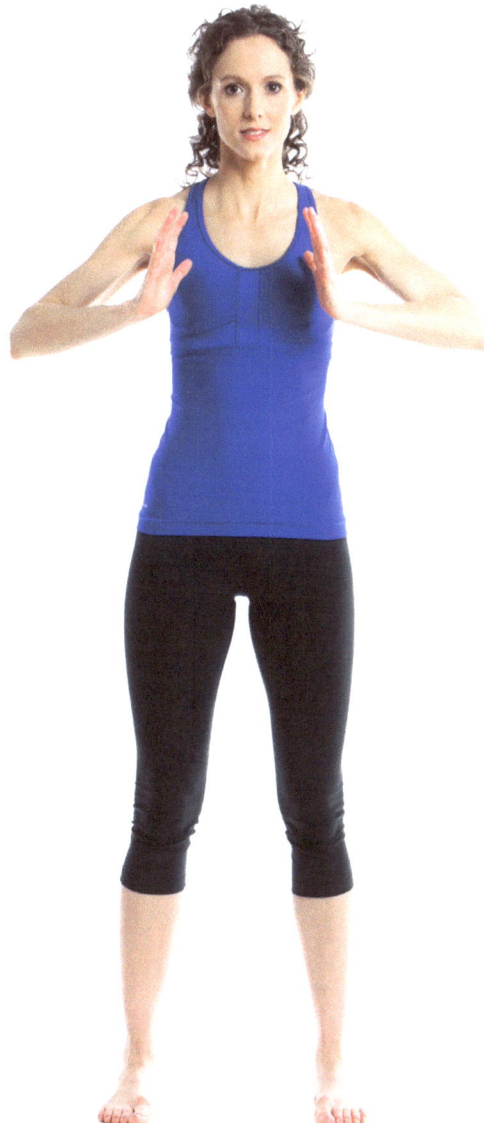

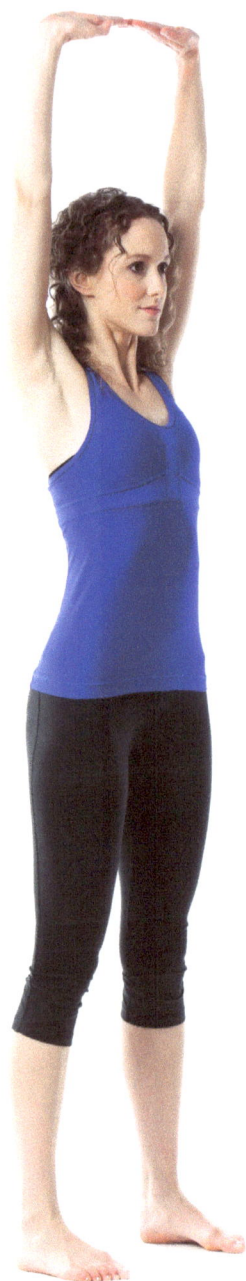

A

Stand straight with your feet shoulder width apart, knees slightly bent, and arms straight up.

Flatten your hands with your palms up and touch your fingertips together. **Inhale**.

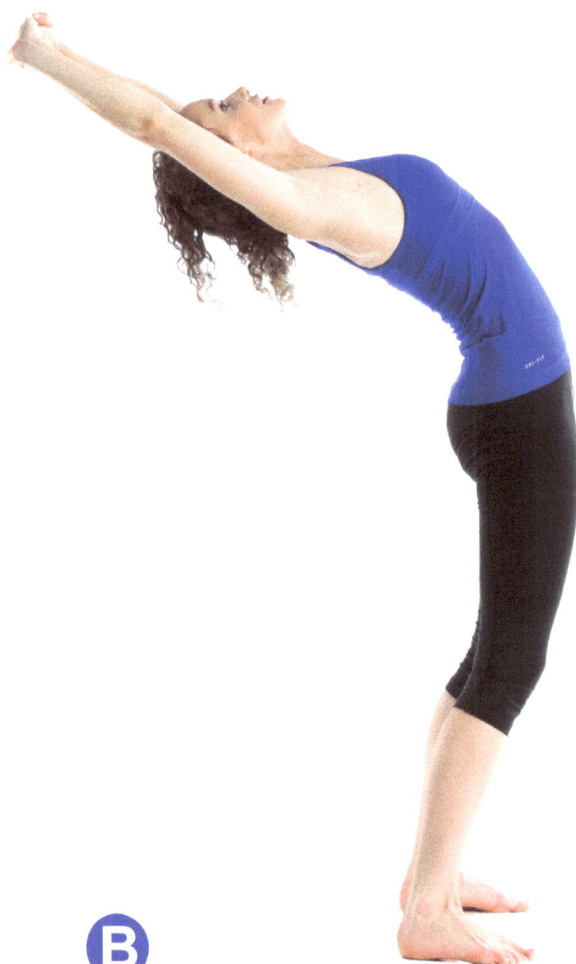

B

Exhale as you bend backward for a stomach stretch and tense your core and glutes to keep your back and body stable.

Hold position **B** on each inhalation and tense harder while bending farther back on each exhalation.

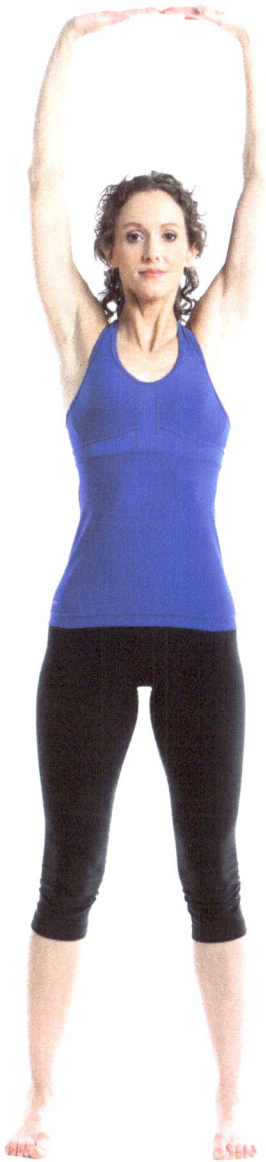

A

Stand straight with your feet shoulder width apart, knees slightly bent, and arms straight up.

Flatten your hands with your palms up and touch your fingertips together.
Inhale.

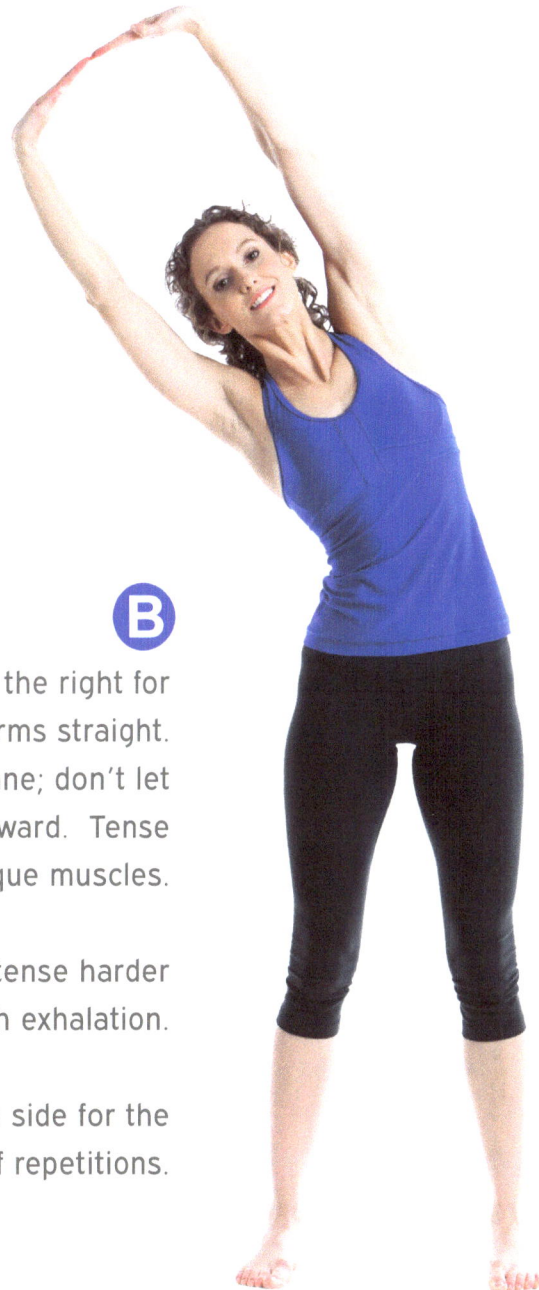

B

Exhale as you bend over to the right for an oblique stretch, keeping your arms straight. Be sure to keep your body in a flat plane; don't let your left shoulder rotate forward or backward. Tense your core, particularly your left oblique muscles.

Hold position **B** on each inhalation and tense harder while bending farther to the right on each exhalation.

Repeat on the opposite side for the same number of repetitions.

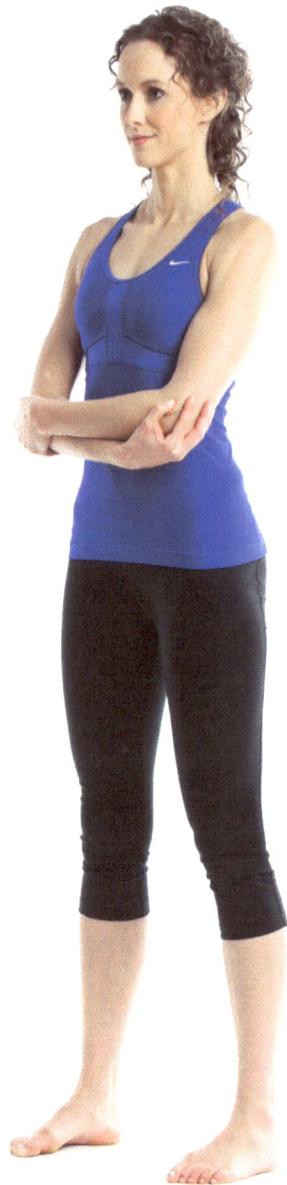

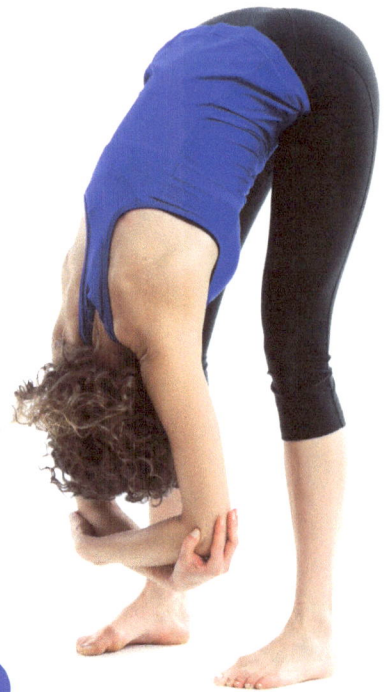

A

Stand straight with your feet shoulder width apart, knees slightly bent. Clasp your elbows.
Inhale.

B

Exhale as you bend forward with a flat back and bring your elbows as close to the floor as possible.

Tense the hamstrings. If you struggle to isolate the hamstring tension, tense your entire thigh and your hamstrings will engage.

Hold position **B** on each inhalation and tense harder while bending farther forward on each exhalation.

Variation:

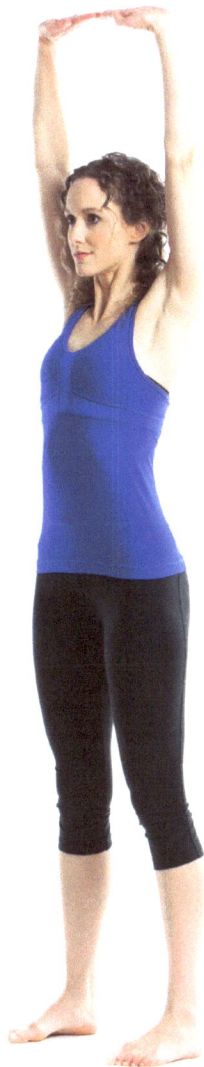

1.1

Use the hand and arm positions of #5 / #6.

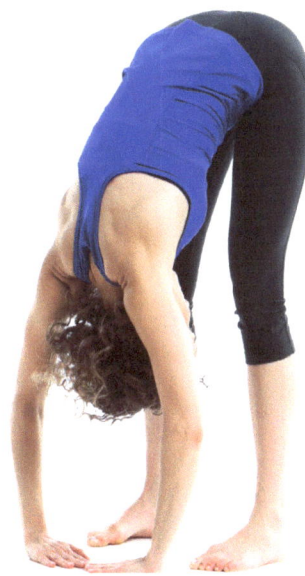

1.2

Bend forward with a straight spine and bring your hands as close to the floor as possible.

A

Stand straight with your feet shoulder width apart, knees slightly bent, and arms straight out front at shoulder height.

Flatten your hands with your palms facing the floor. **Inhale**.

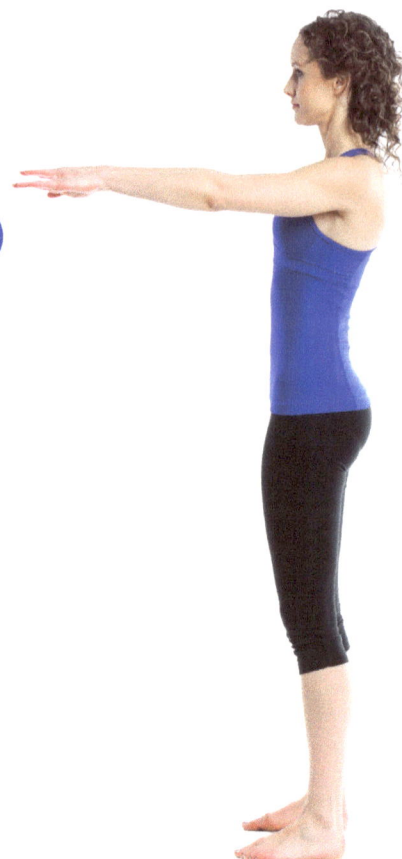

This exercise does not follow the typical I Chin Ching breathing pattern.

B

Hold your breath as you drop your shoulders. Your palms may face slightly forward as a result of the shoulder drop. Relax and **exhale** normally.

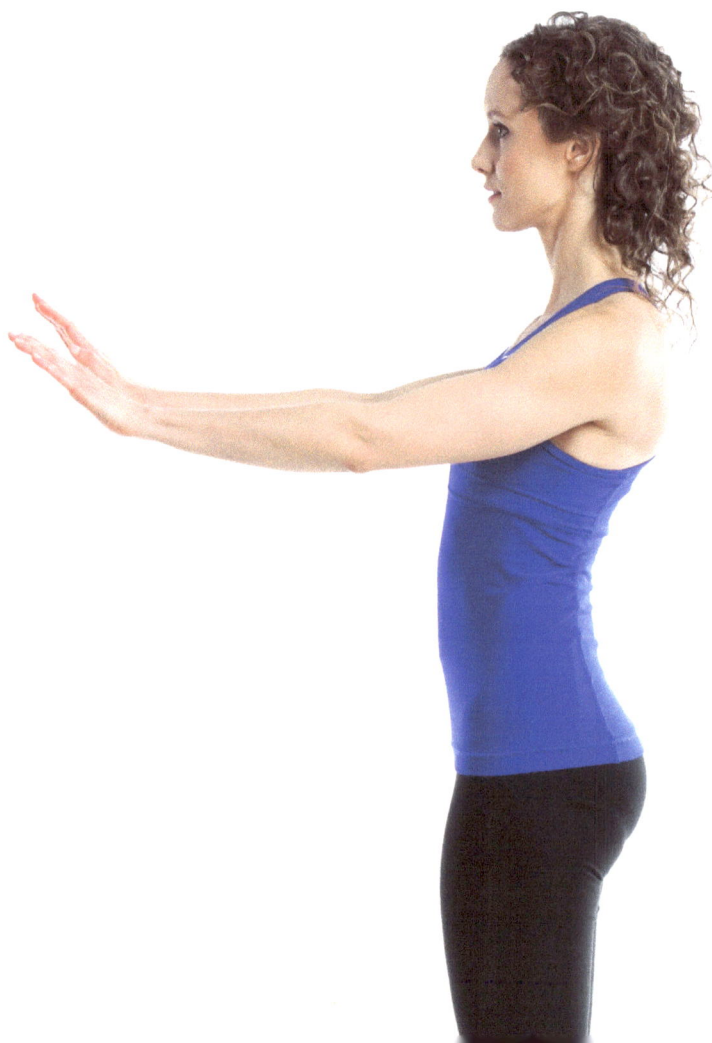

Repeat **A** and **B** without any focus on tension or without increasing the intensity of the exercise with each repetition.

A

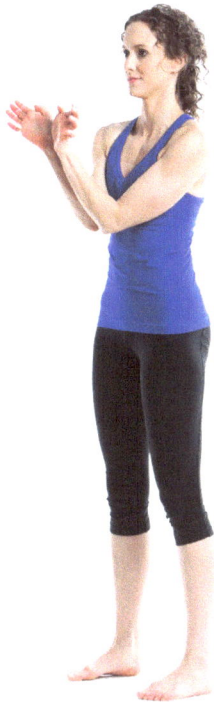

Stand straight with your feet shoulder width apart, knees slightly bent, and your arms in front of your chest with your elbows touching and palms out.

B

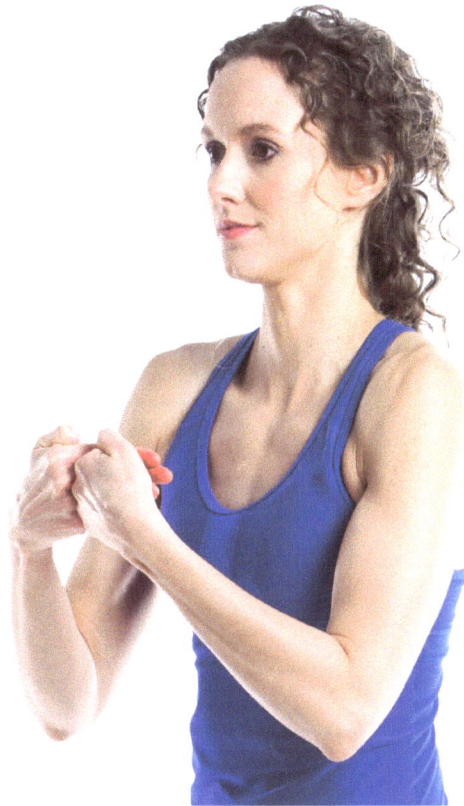

Inhale as you curl your fingers and hands in so that the backs of your knuckles touch with thumbs up.

This exercise does not follow the typical I Chin Ching breathing pattern.

C

Hold your breath as you bring your knuckles to touch your chest.

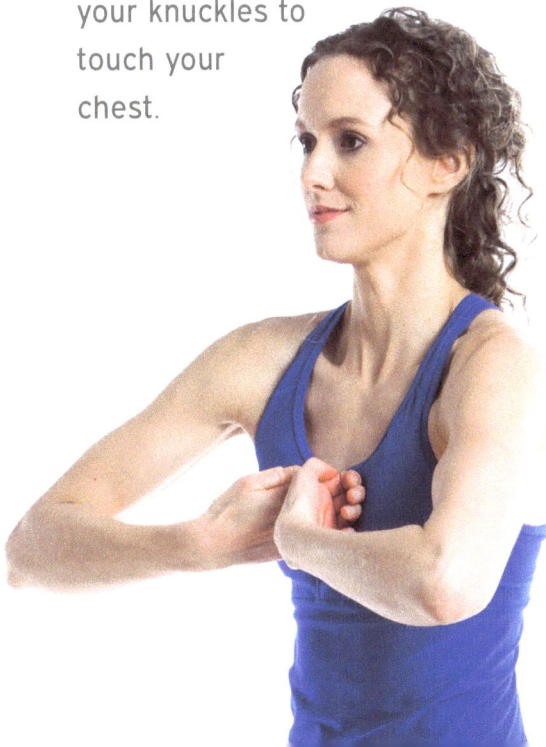

D

Continue holding your breath as you bring your hands up and drop your elbows until they touch again. **Exhale** normally.

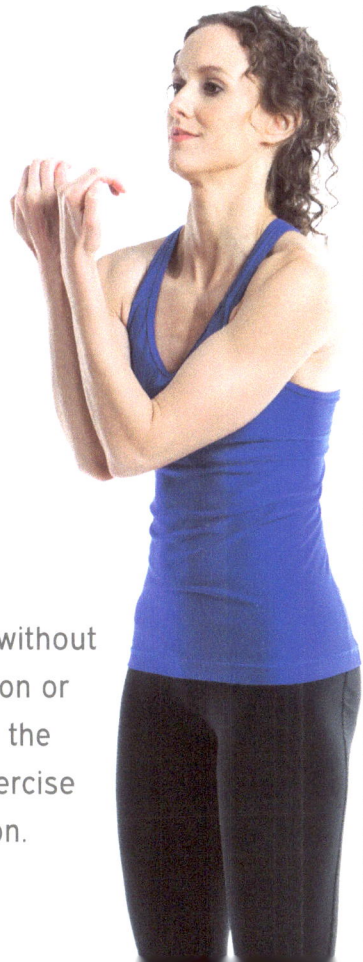

Repeat each step without any focus on tension or without increasing the intensity of the exercise with each repetition.

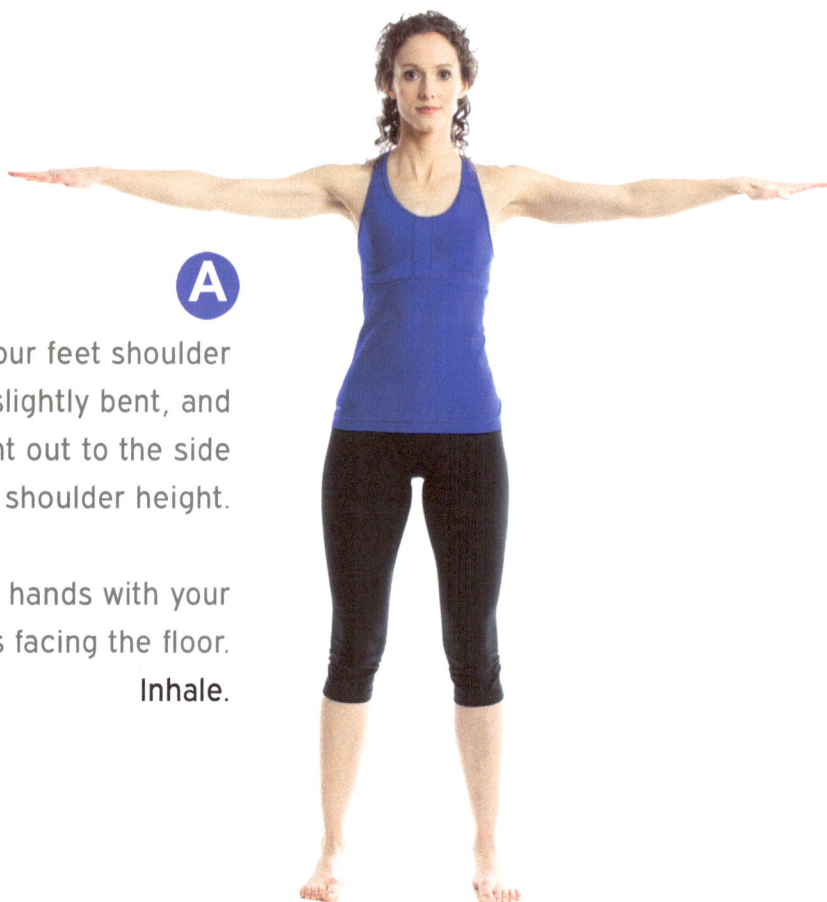

A

Stand straight with your feet shoulder width apart, knees slightly bent, and arms straight out to the side at shoulder height.

Flatten your hands with your palms facing the floor.
Inhale.

This exercise does not follow the typical I Chin Ching breathing pattern.

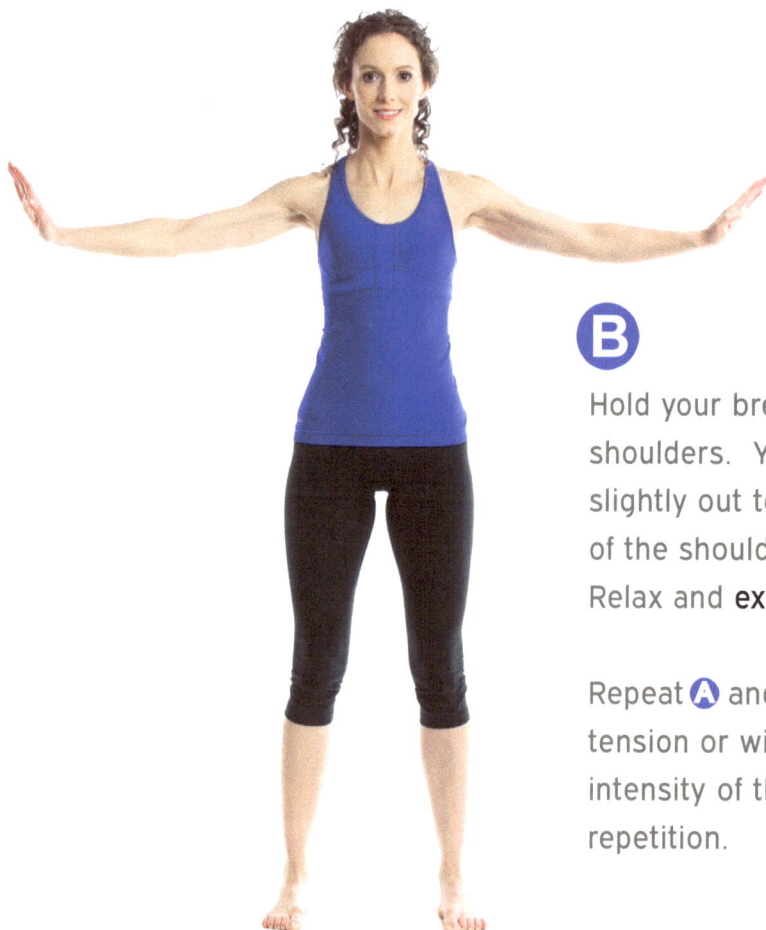

B

Hold your breath as you drop your shoulders. Your palms may face slightly out to the side as a result of the shoulder drop.
Relax and **exhale** normally.

Repeat **A** and **B** without any focus on tension or without increasing the intensity of the exercise with each repetition.

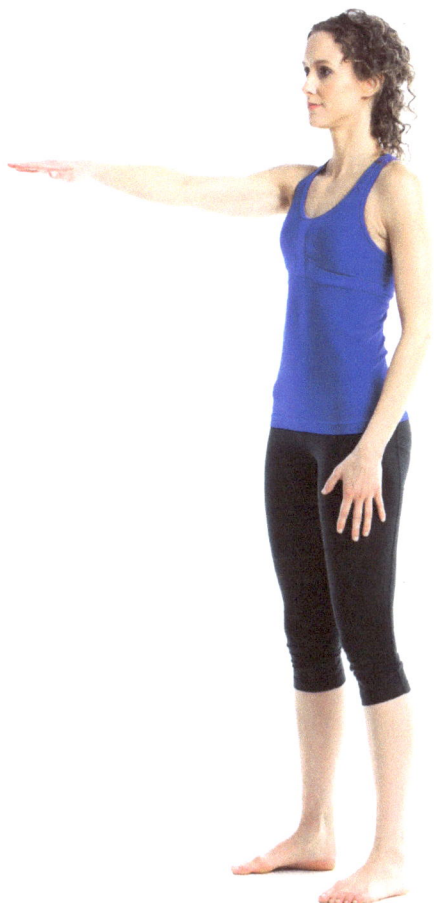

A

Stand straight with your feet shoulder width apart, knees slightly bent, and right arm straight out front at shoulder height.

Flatten your hand with your palm facing the floor. **Inhale**.

This exercise does not follow the typical I Chin Ching breathing pattern. It is just like #8 but one arm at a time.

B

Hold your breath as you drop your shoulder. Your palm may face slightly forward as a result of the shoulder drop. Relax and **exhale** normally.

Repeat **A** and **B** without any focus on tension or without increasing the intensity of the exercise with each repetition.

Repeat on the opposite side for the same number of repetitions.

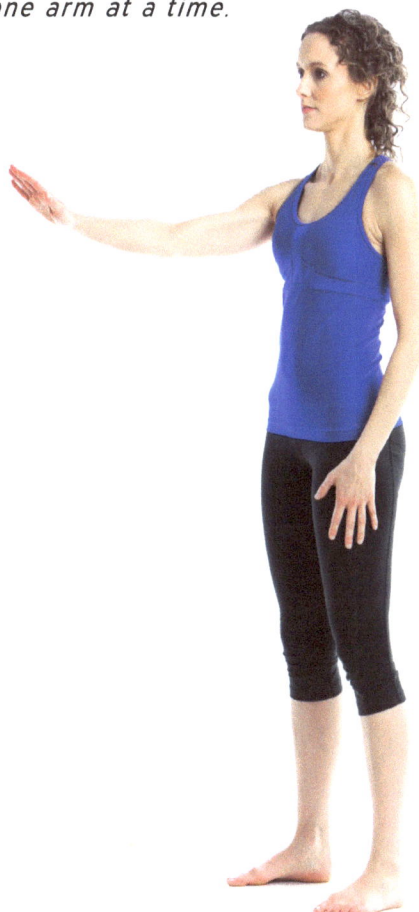

A

Stand straight with your feet shoulder width apart, knees slightly bent, and left arm straight out to the side at shoulder height.

Flatten your hand with your palm facing the floor. **Inhale**.

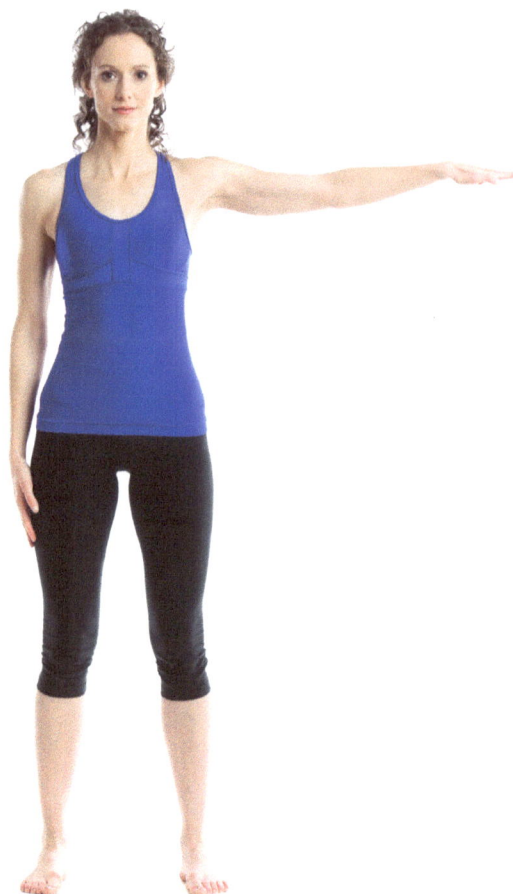

This exercise does not follow the typical I Chin Ching breathing pattern. It is just like #10 but one arm at a time.

B

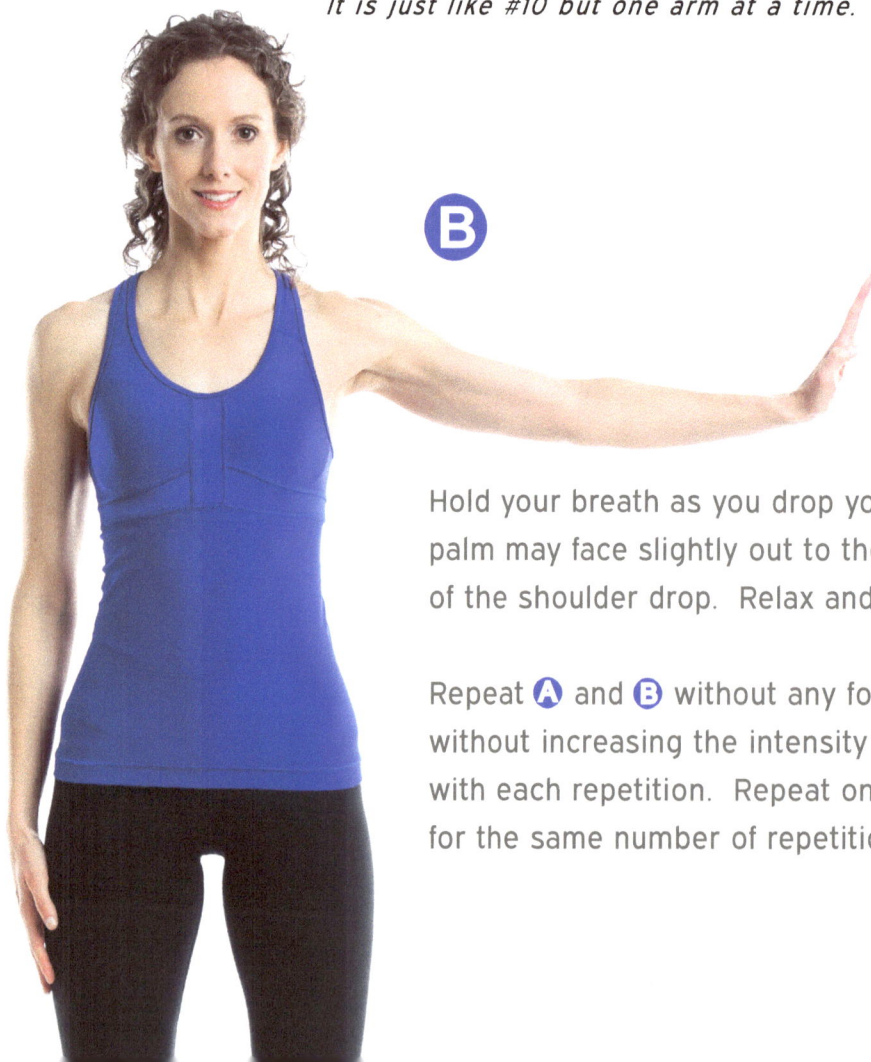

Hold your breath as you drop your shoulder. Your palm may face slightly out to the side as a result of the shoulder drop. Relax and **exhale** normally.

Repeat **A** and **B** without any focus on tension or without increasing the intensity of the exercise with each repetition. Repeat on the opposite side for the same number of repetitions.

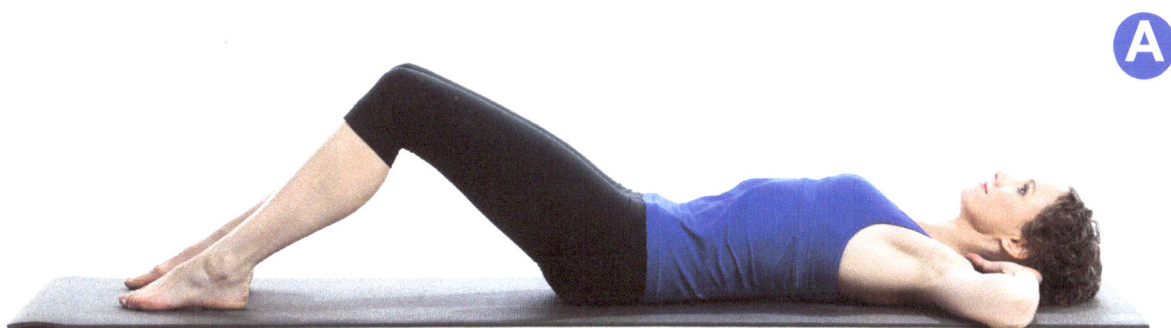

Lie down on your back with your knees bent and feet flat on the floor.

Touch your fingertips to the back of your head with your elbows out to the side.
Inhale.

B

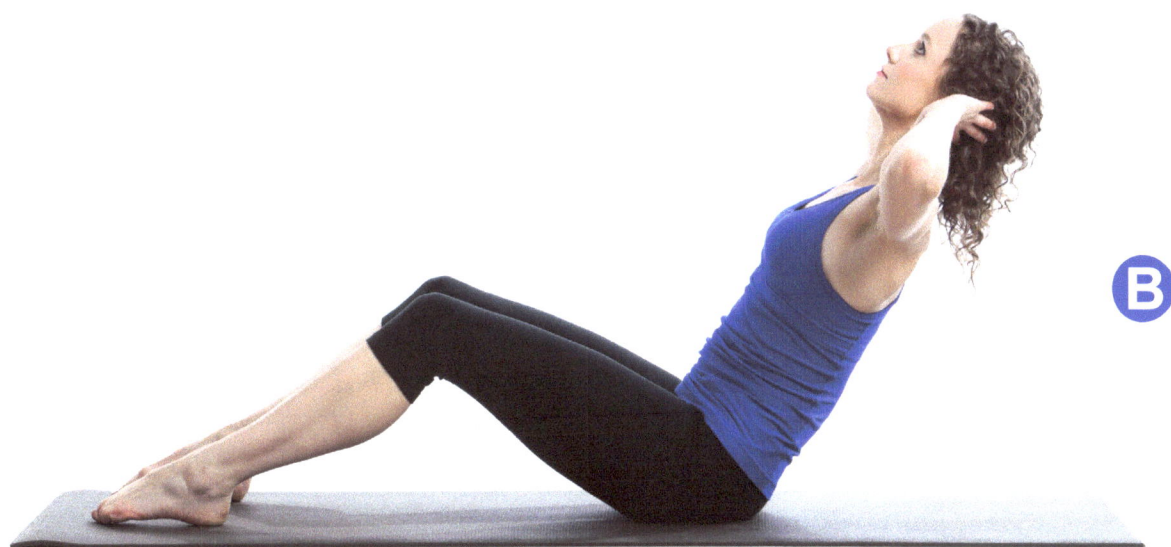

Exhale as you sit up at a 45 degree angle and tense your upper stomach muscles. Keep your chest and chin lifted with your spine straight.
Look towards the ceiling.

Hold position B on each inhalation and tense harder on each exhalation.

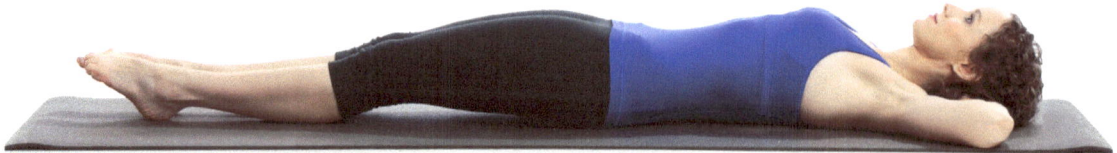

A Lie down on your back with your legs straight out in front of you.
Rest your head on your hands.
Inhale.

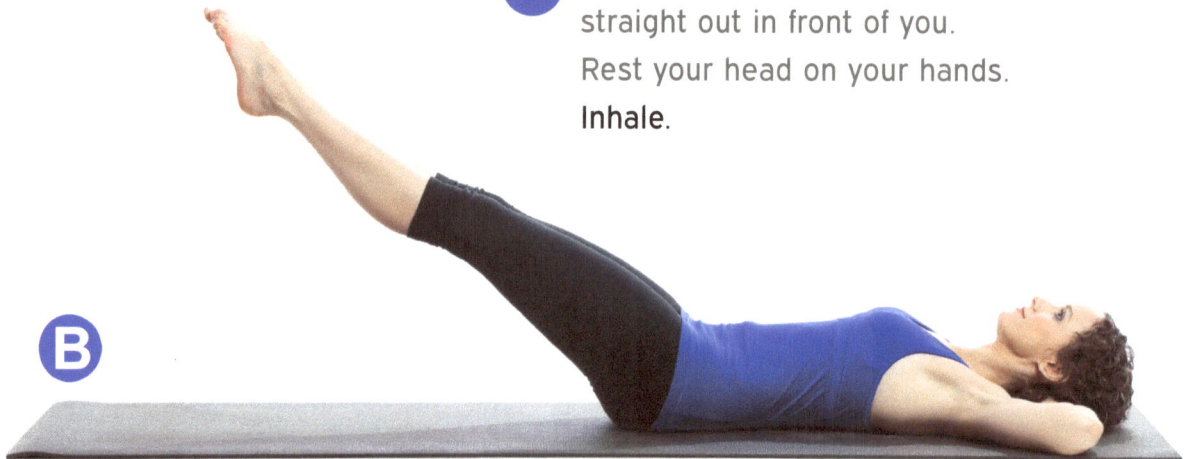

B

Exhale as you lift both legs to a 45 degree angle and tense your lower stomach muscles.

Be sure to keep your lower back pressed to the floor so there is no space between your back and the floor.

Hold position **B** on each inhalation and tense harder on each exhalation.

Variations:

It can be difficult to hold your legs at a 45 degree angle without arching your lower back. If your lower back is arched, you won't get the full tension in your stomach muscles and you run the risk of straining your lower back.

Try these variations if your lower back is arching.

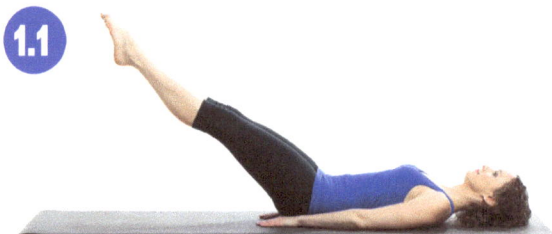

1.1

Place your hands behind your glutes. Keep your hands there for every repetition.

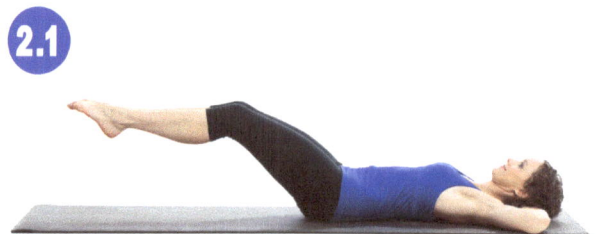

2.1

Bend your knees as much as you need to keep your lower back pressed to the floor.

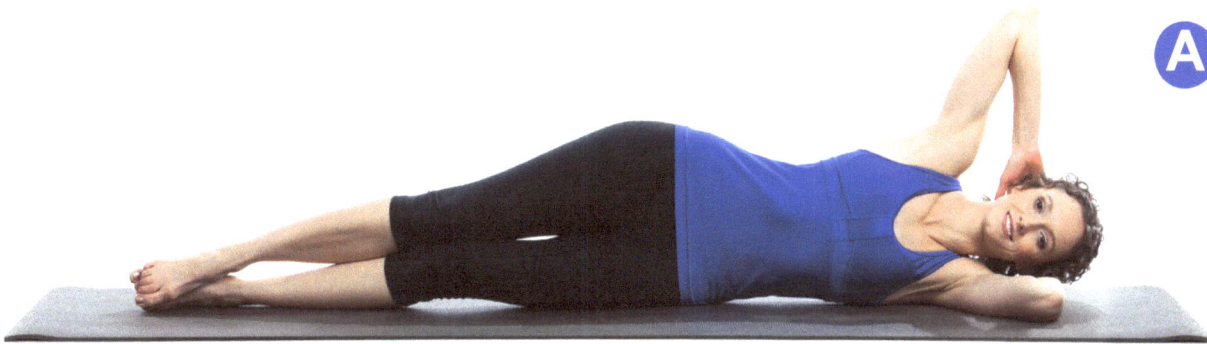

Lie on your left side with your body straight so that your shoulders, hips, legs, and feet are stacked on top of each other.

Touch your fingertips to the back of your head with your elbows out to the side. **Inhale**.

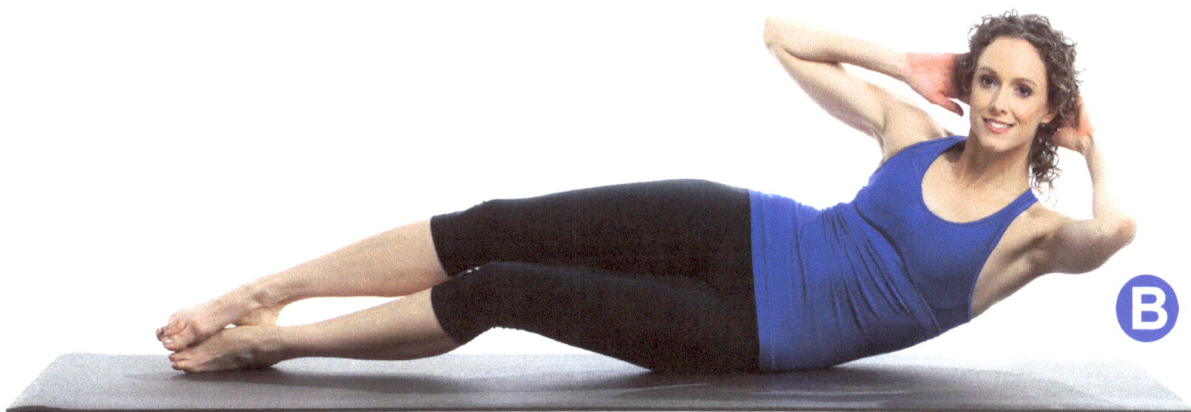

B

Exhale as you lift your chest and head up to a 45 degree angle and tense your right oblique muscles. Be sure to remain completely on your side; don't fall back on your left glute.

Hold position B on each inhalation and tense harder on each exhalation. Repeat on the opposite side for the same number of repetitions.

A

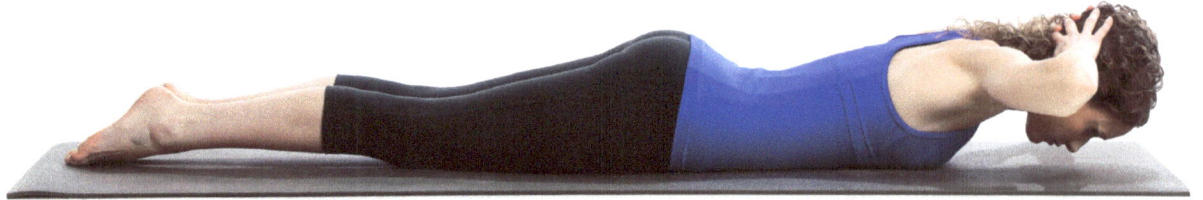

Lie face down on the floor with your legs straight out behind you.

Touch your fingertips to the back of your head with your elbows out to the side. **Inhale**.

B

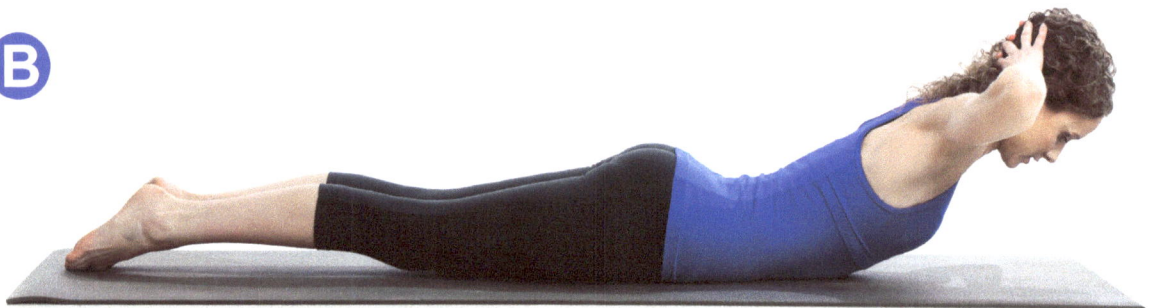

Exhale as you lift your chest off the floor and tense your lower back and in between your shoulder blades. Keep your face towards the floor.

Hold position **B** on each inhalation and lift higher and tense harder on each exhalation.

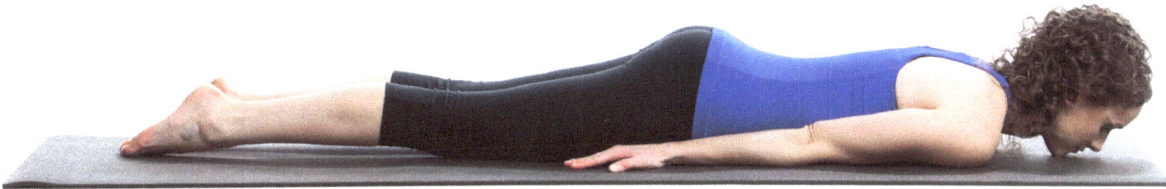

Lie face down on the floor with your legs straight out behind you.

Place your arms straight by your sides with your palms on the floor. **Inhale**.

B

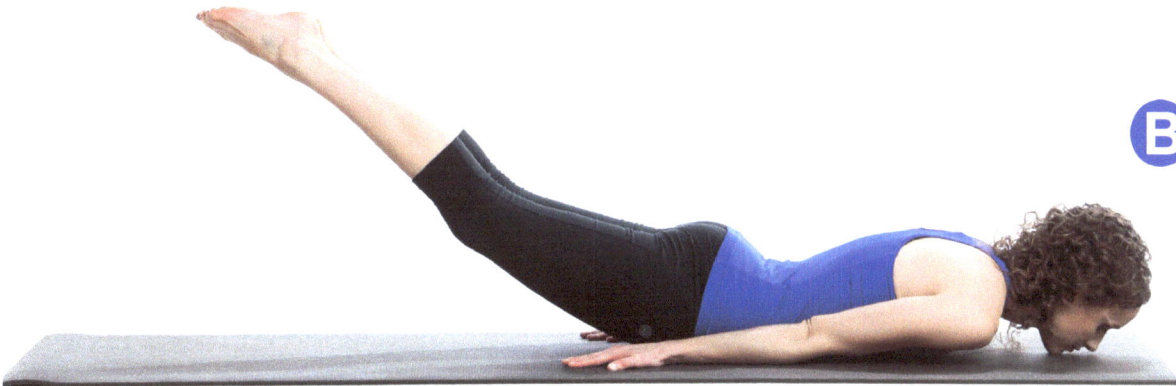

Exhale as you lift your thighs off the floor and tense your glutes and hamstrings. Be sure to keep your knees straight.

Hold position B on each inhalation and lift higher and tense harder on each exhalation.

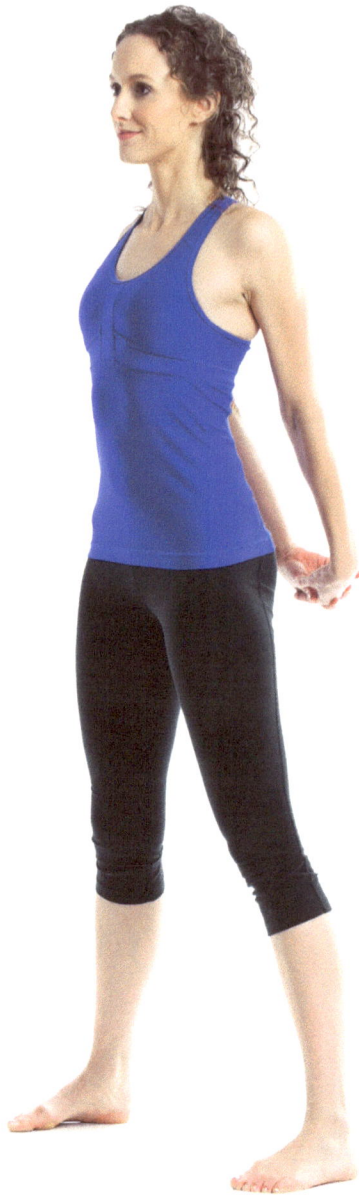

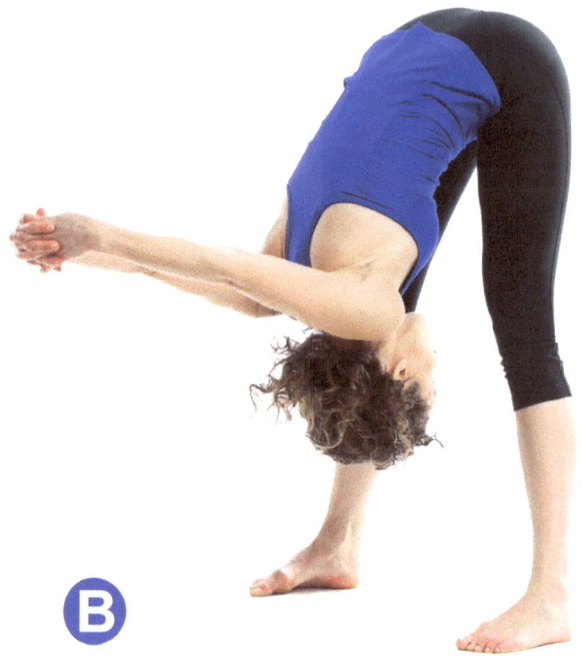

A

Stand straight with your feet wider than shoulder width apart and knees slightly bent.

Clasp your hands behind your back while keeping your arms straight. **Inhale**.

B

Exhale as you bend forward with a straight spine and stretch your arms as high up and over your back as possible for a shoulder stretch.

Hold position **B** on each inhalation and stretch farther on each exhalation.

A

Stand straight with your feet shoulder width apart, knees slightly bent.

Place your left arm behind your back with your palm out and place your right hand behind your head. **Inhale.**

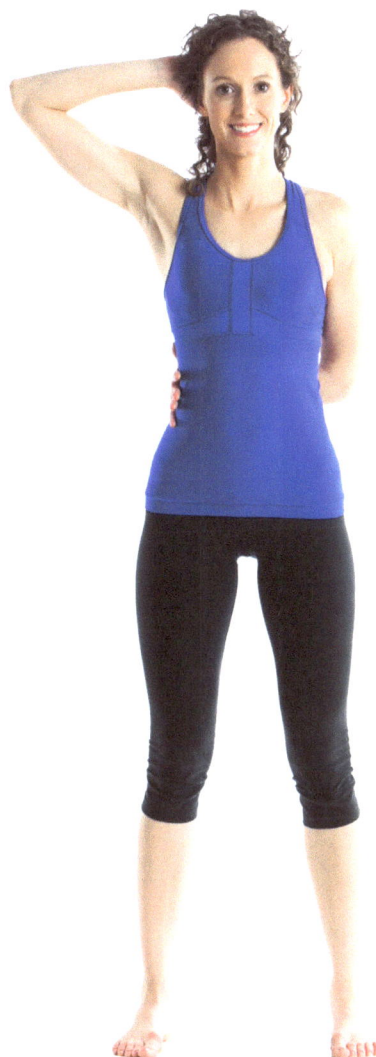

B

Exhale as you twist your body to the left for a spinal twist stretch.

Hold position **B** on each inhalation and stretch farther on each exhalation.

Repeat on the opposite side for the same number of repetitions.

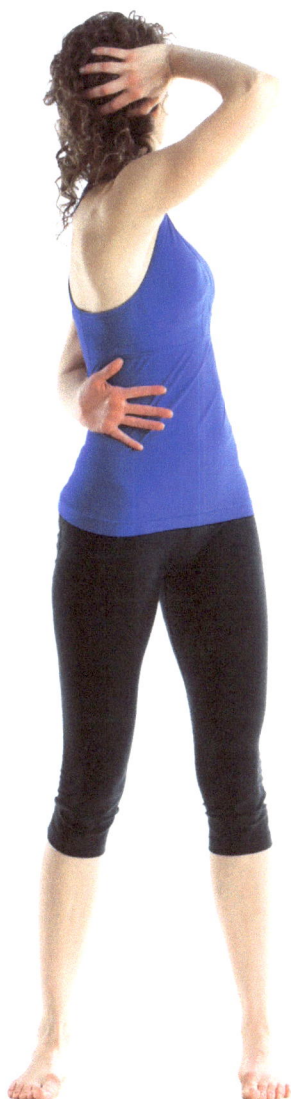

20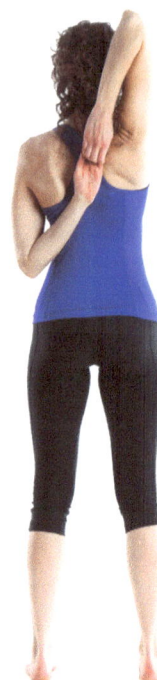

A

Stand straight with your feet shoulder width apart, knees slightly bent. Place your right hand on your upper back, with your palm touching your back and your elbow pointing up.

Bring your left hand behind your back with your palm out and clasp your fingers.
Inhale.

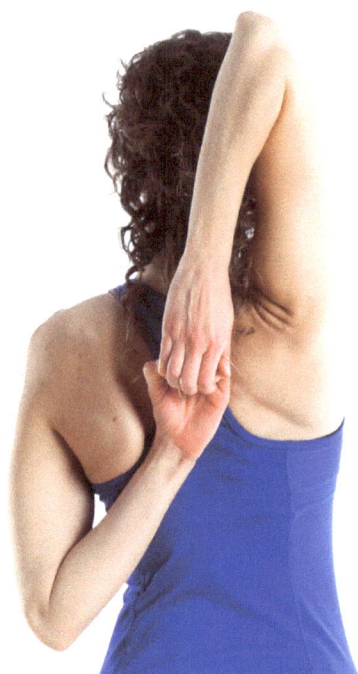

B

Exhale as you use your left hand to pull your right hand down for a triceps stretch. Be sure to keep your chest and chin up; don't let the elbow of the right arm press your head forward.

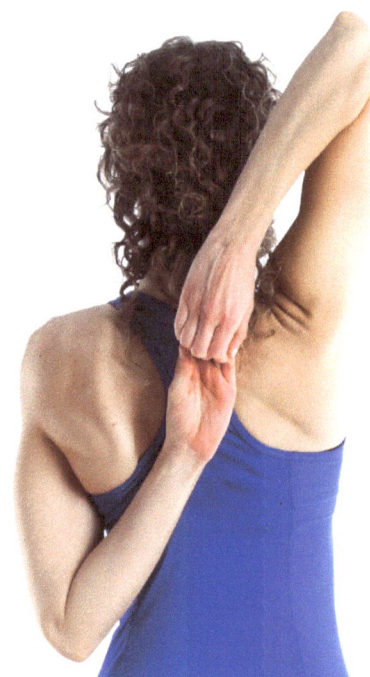

C

Hold position **B** on the inhalation and on the next exhalation use your right hand to pull your left hand up for a shoulder stretch as seen above, in position **C**.

Do the same number of triceps stretches and shoulder stretches, then repeat on the opposite arm for the same number of repetitions.

Variations:

1.1

Use your left arm to pull your elbow in for a triceps stretch.

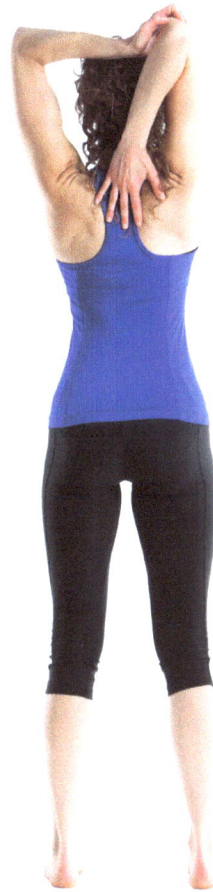

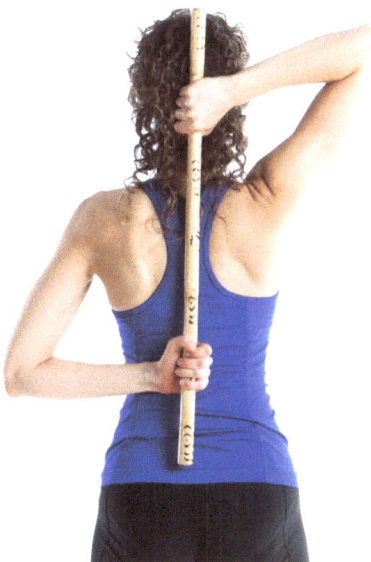

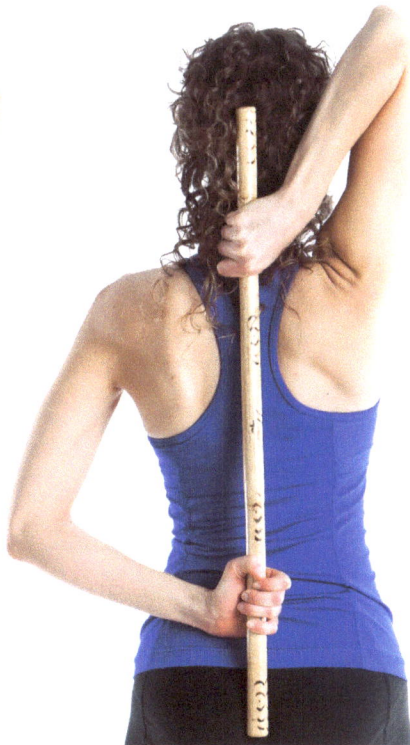

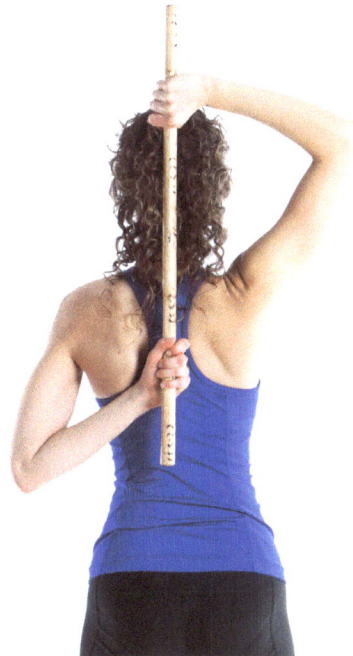

2.1

Use a towel, belt, or short stick to assist the triceps and shoulder stretches.

A

21 Sit down with a straight spine and extend your right leg directly in front of you.

Bring your left foot to the outside of your right leg, as high up the leg as you can.

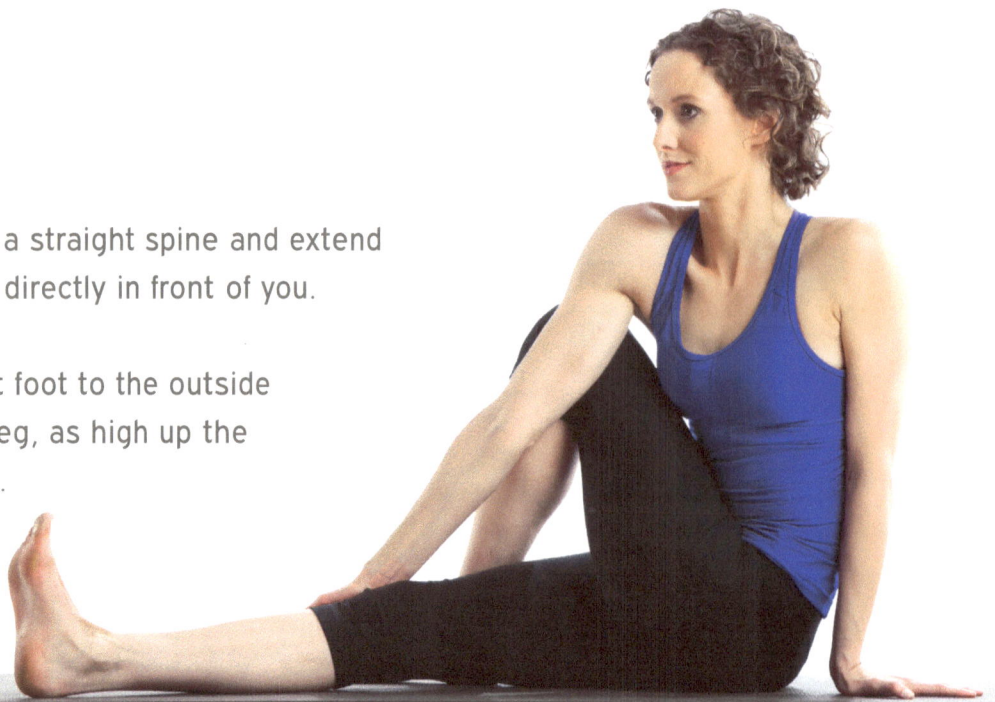

Reach around your left knee with your right arm and clasp underneath the right knee.

Plant your left hand directly behind your hip with your palm on the floor.
Inhale.

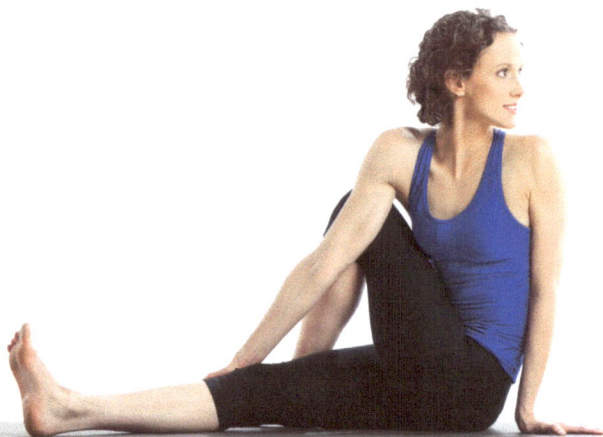

B

Exhale as you twist your body and head to the left for a spinal twist stretch.

Hold position **B** on each inhalation and stretch farther on each exhalation. Repeat on the opposite side for the same number of repetitions.

Variation:

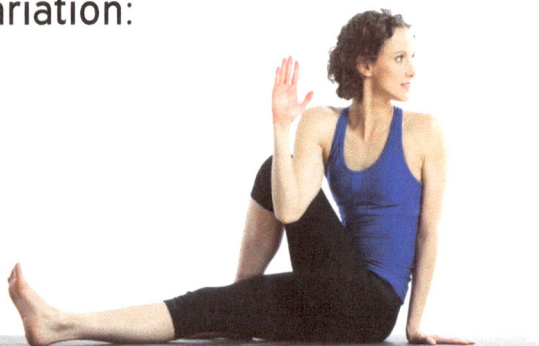

1.1

Reach around your left knee with your right arm and brace your right elbow against the outside of the left knee.

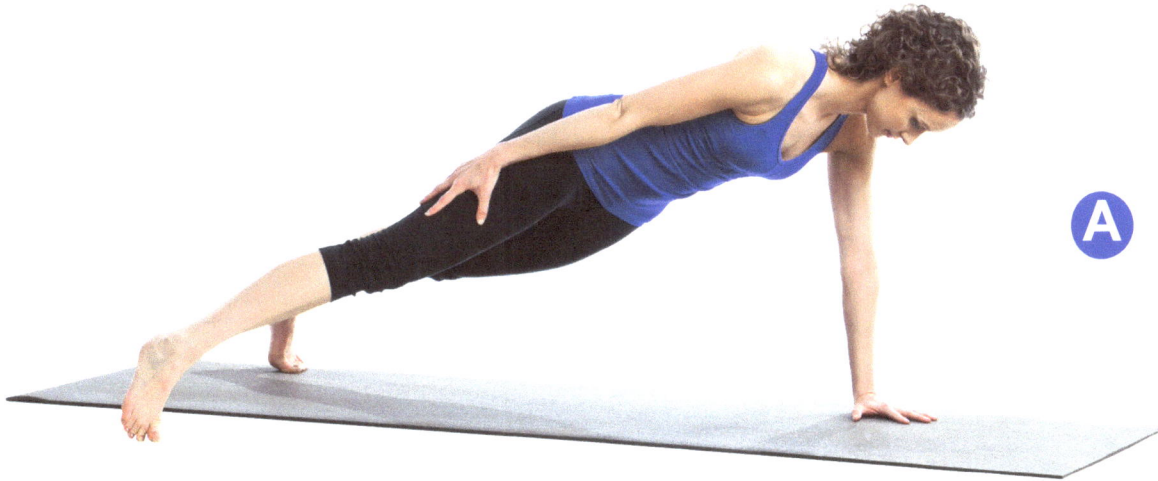

Start in a high pushup position with your hands directly underneath your shoulders. Twist your body slightly to the right and brace your right hand on the outside of your right leg.

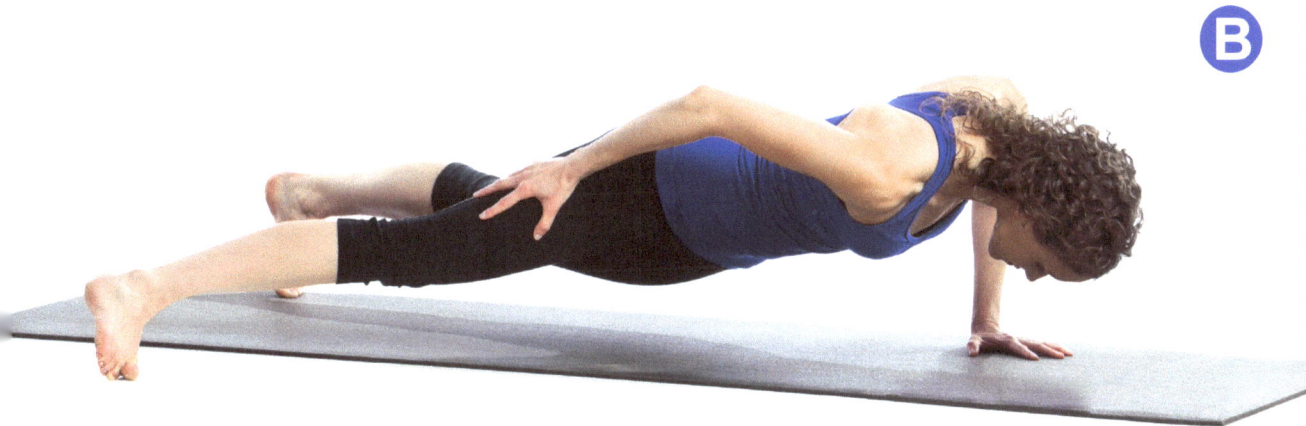

B

Inhale as you lower your body into a one-arm pushup.

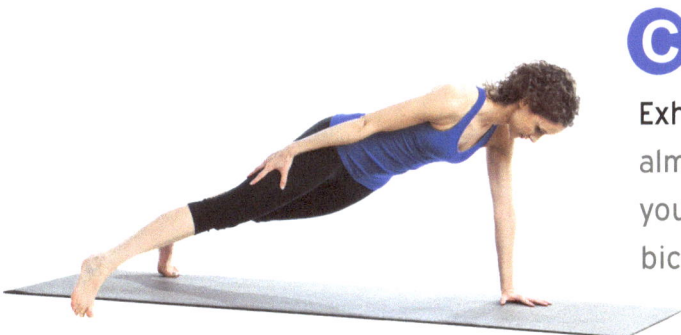

C

Exhale as you straighten your left arm almost all the way, without locking your elbow, and tense your left biceps and chest muscles.

Lower back down to a one-arm pushup on the inhalation and straighten your arm and tense harder on each exhalation. You may need to adjust the width of your feet to achieve the one-arm pushup.

Repeat on the opposite side for the same number of repetitions.

Variations:

1.1

Drop to your knees for the one-arm pushup.

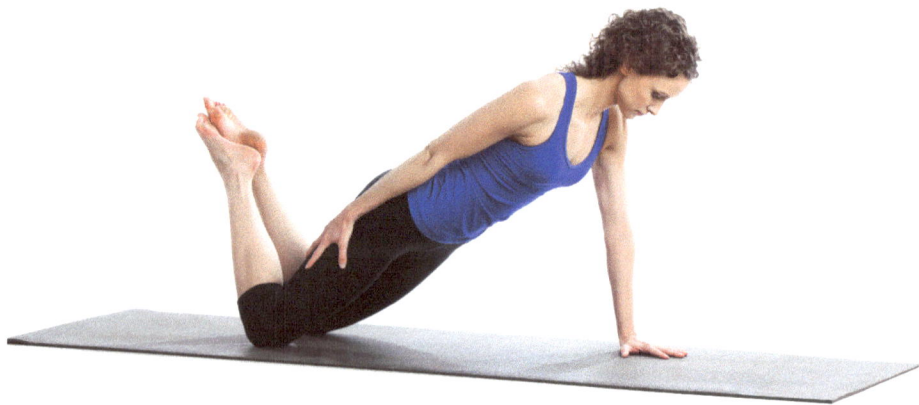

1.2

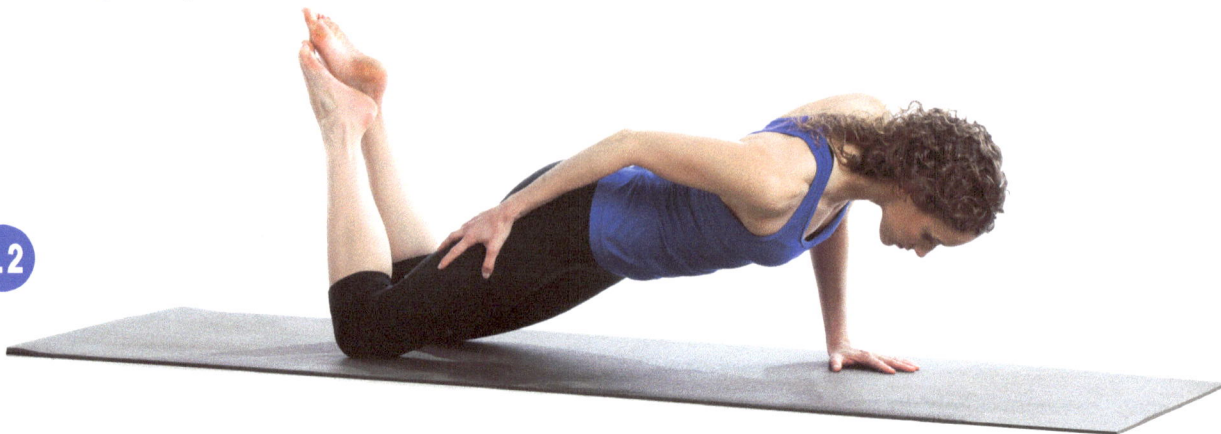

2.1

Use both arms for the pushup then gradually move your right hand away from your left hand to put more effort on the left arm as you build strength.

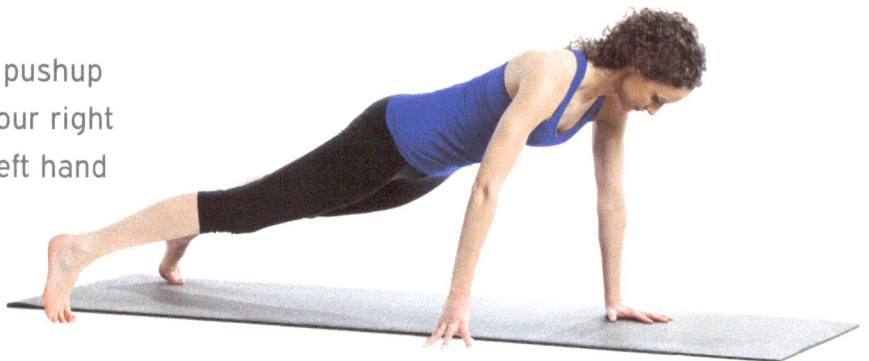

2.2

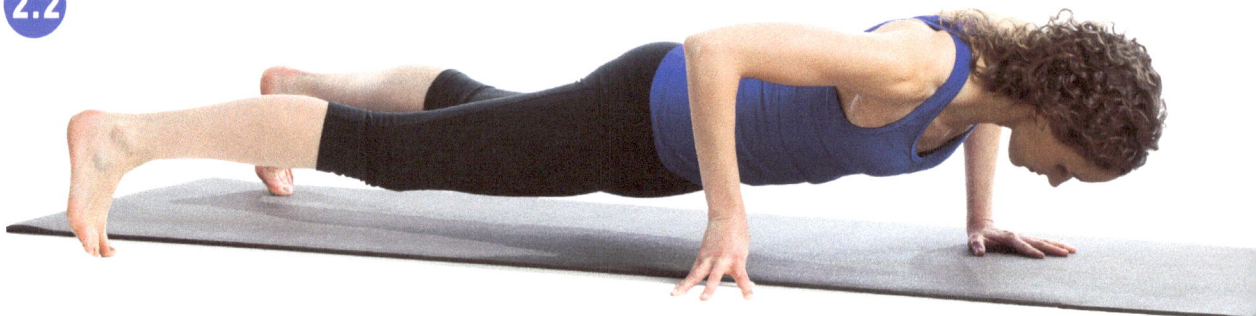

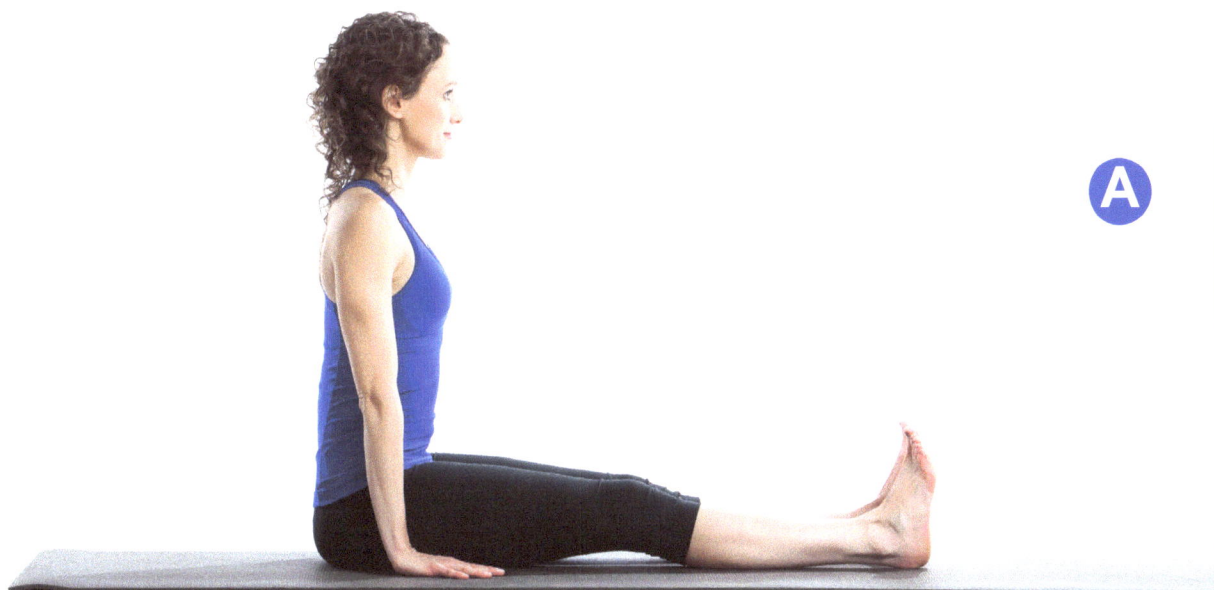

Sit down with a straight spine with your legs straight in front of you.

Place your palms on the floor, slightly in front of your hips, with your fingers pointing towards your feet.
Inhale.

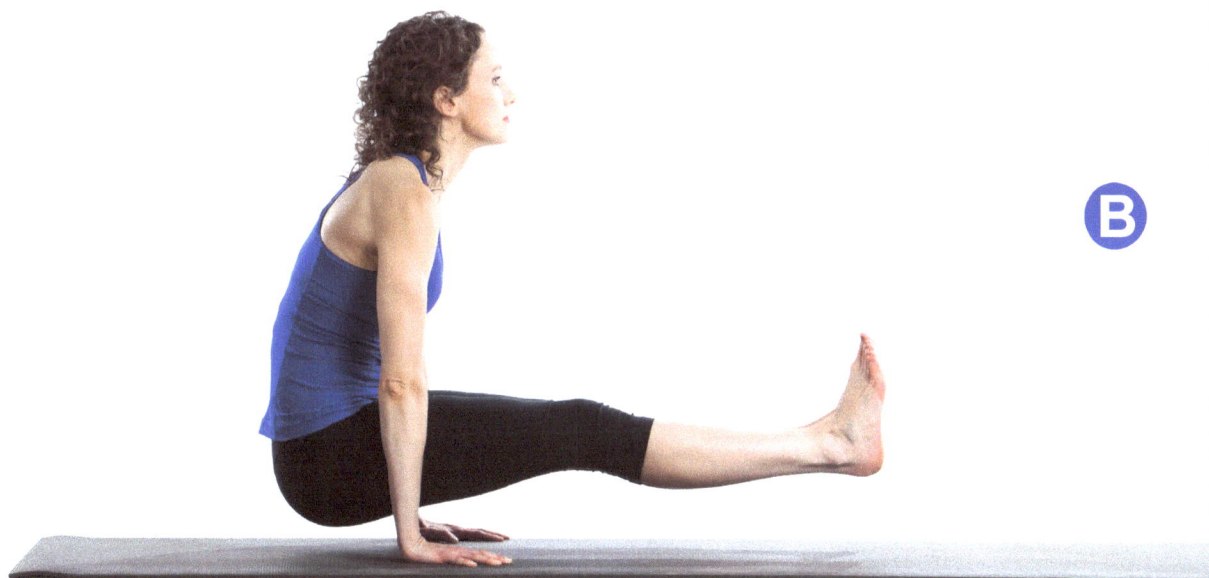

B

Exhale as you press your hips, legs, and feet off the floor and tense your lower stomach muscles and quads.

Hold position **B** on each inhalation and tense harder and press higher on the exhalation.

Variations:

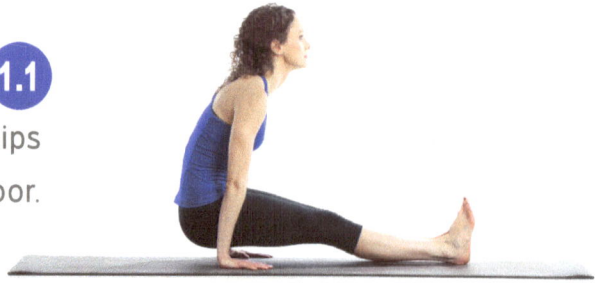

1.1 Press only your hips and legs off the floor.

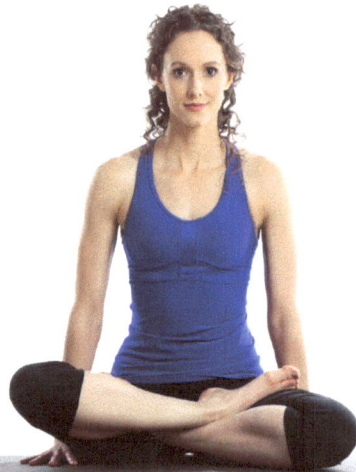

2.1

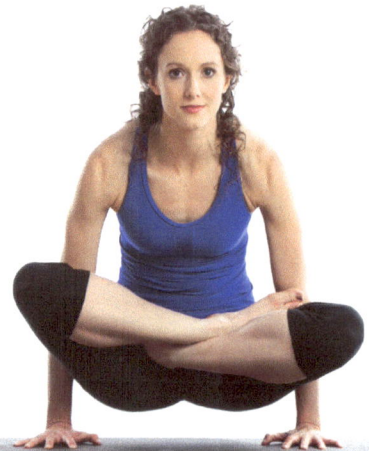

2.2

Sit in a cross legged or lotus position and press your legs off the floor. Gradually extend your legs as you build strength.

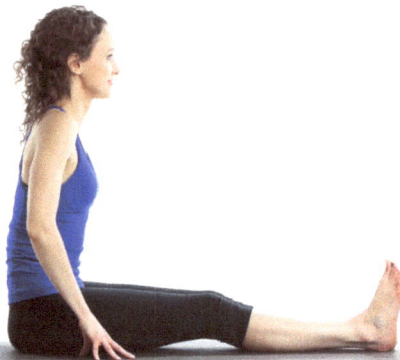

3.1

Use fists or fingertips for the hand position, rather than flat palms.

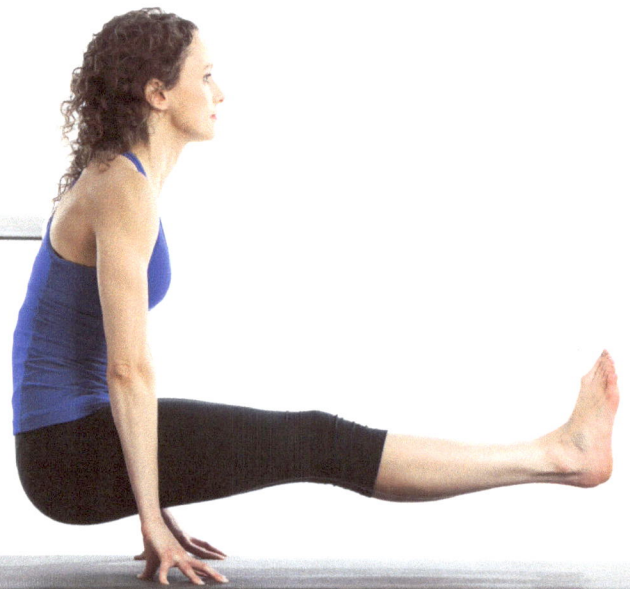

3.2

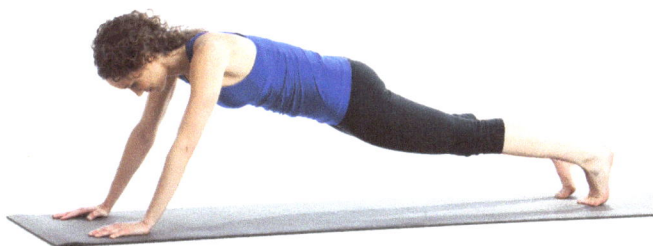

A

Start in a high pushup position with your hands out in front of your body.

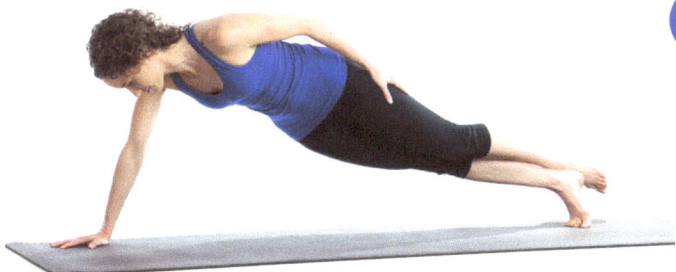

B

Twist your body to the left so that your right hand and right foot touch the floor and cross your left foot behind your right ankle.

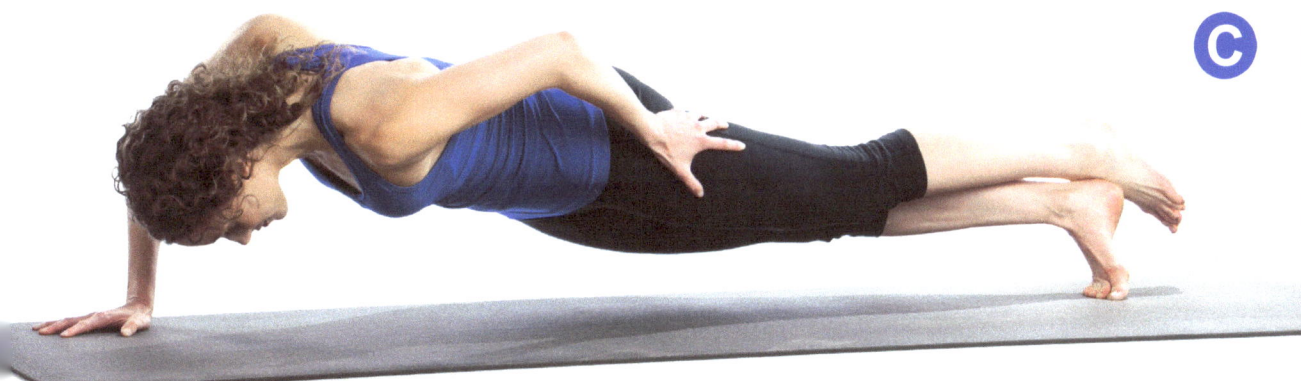

C

Inhale as you lower your body into a one-arm/one-foot pushup.

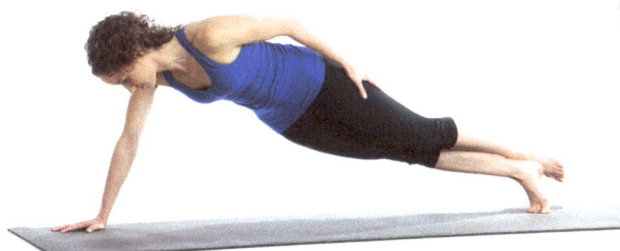

D

Exhale as you straighten your right arm almost all the way, without locking your elbow, and tense your right biceps and chest muscles.

Lower back down to a one-arm/one-foot pushup on each inhalation and straighten your arm and tense harder on each exhalation.

Repeat on the opposite side for the same number of repetitions.

Variations:

1.1

Use both arms for the pushup then gradually move your left hand away from your right hand to put more effort on the right arm as you build strength.

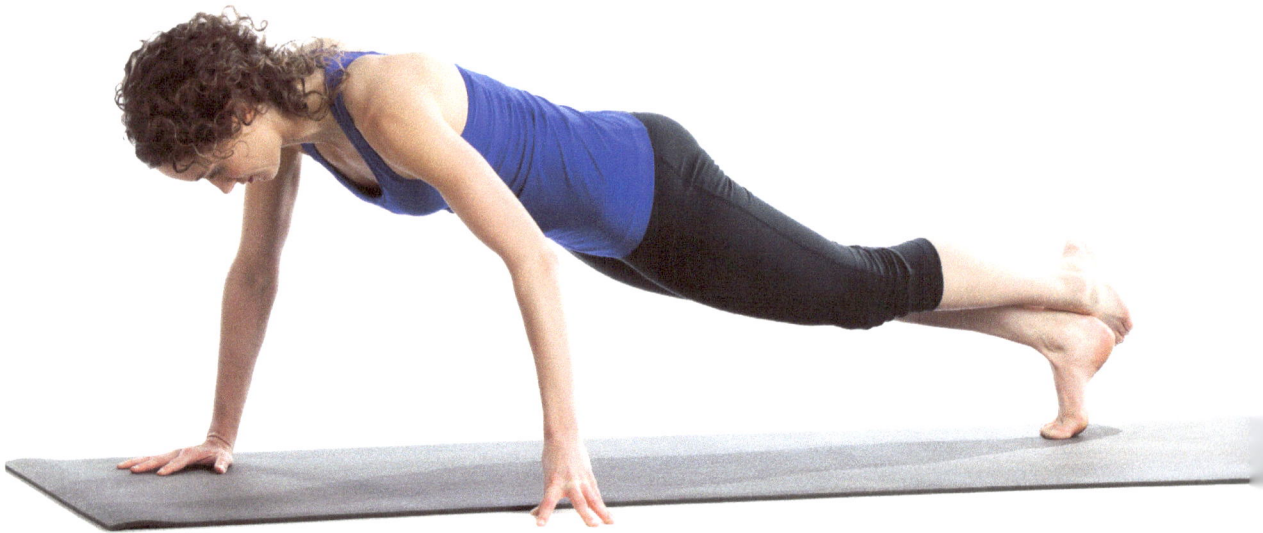

1.2

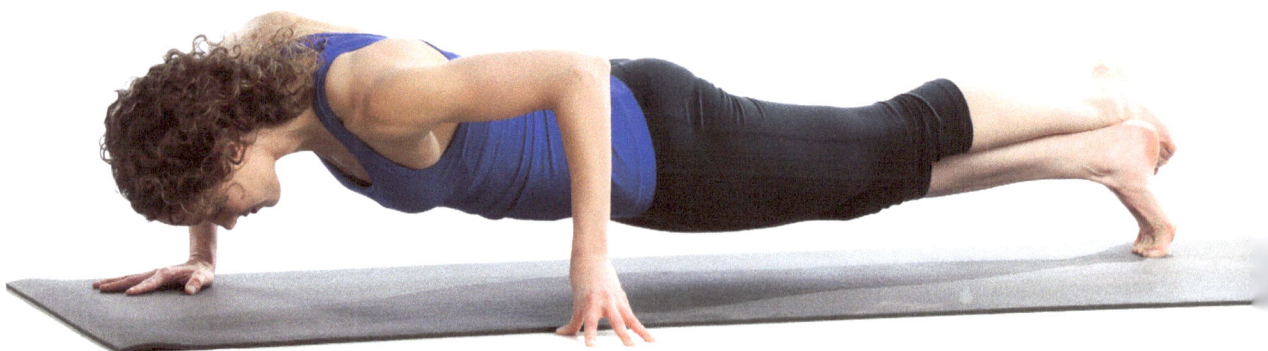

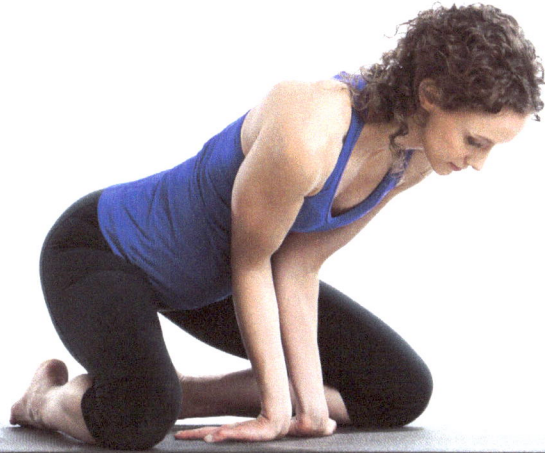

Sit on your feet with your knees spread apart. Press your elbows into your stomach and place your palms on the floor in between your legs so that your fingertips point towards your feet.

Inhale.

B

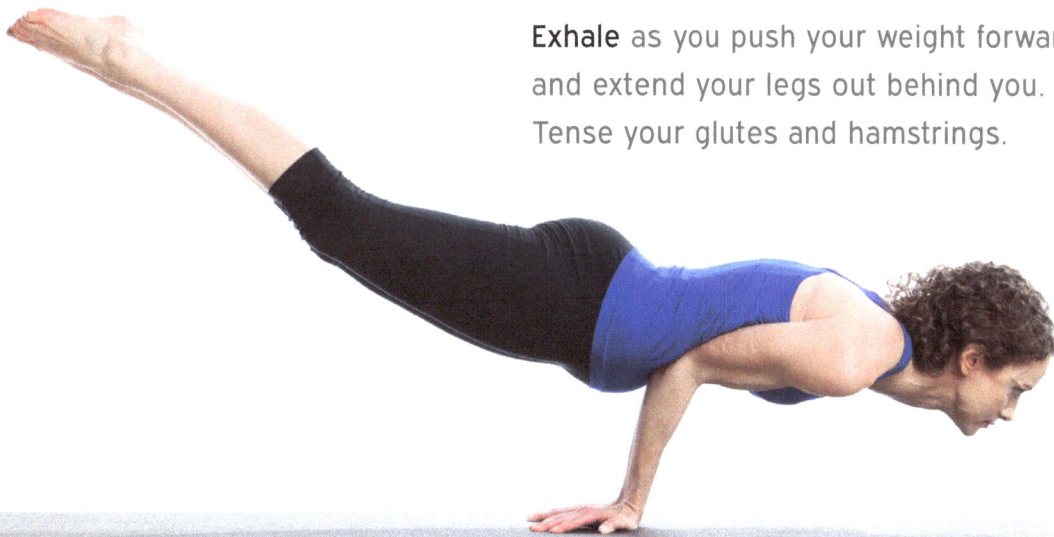

Exhale as you push your weight forward and extend your legs out behind you. Tense your glutes and hamstrings.

Hold position B on each inhalation and tense harder on the exhalation.

Variations:

1.1

Use your head as an extra balance point to help pick your feet up off the floor.

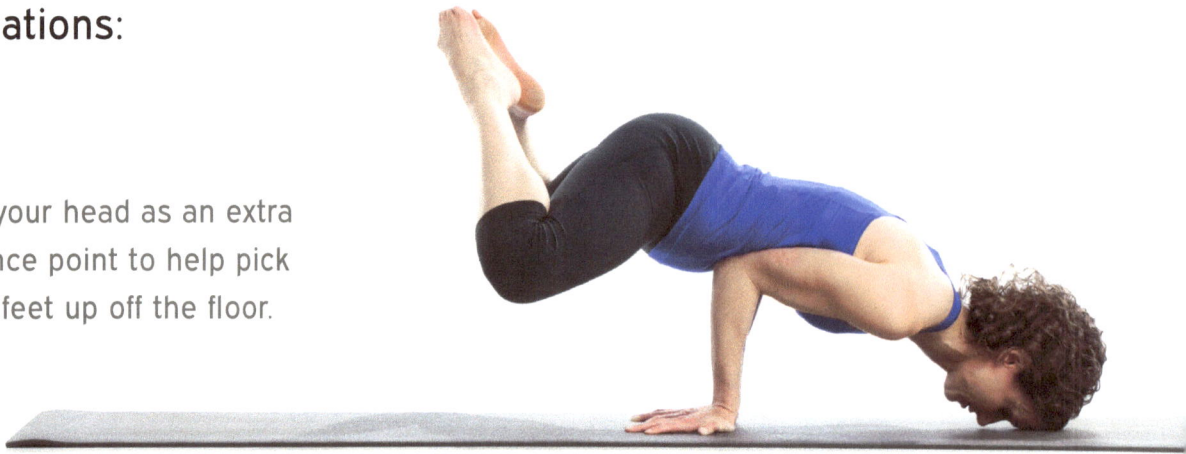

2.1

Keep the knees bent rather than extending the legs out behind you.

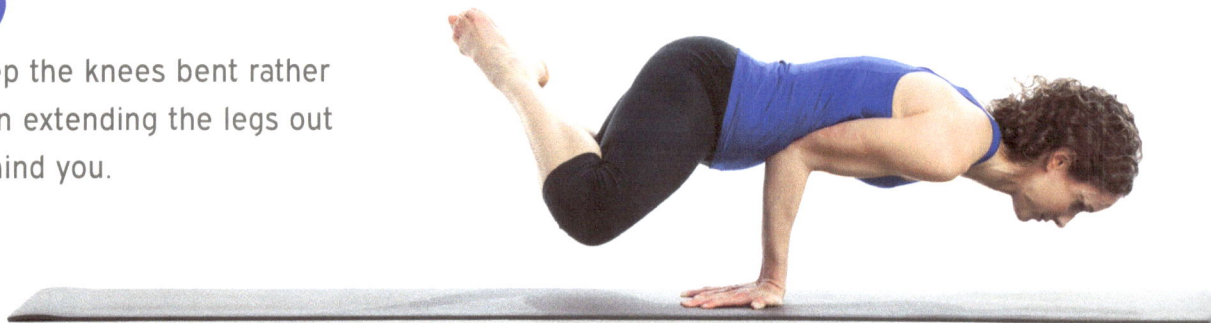

3.1

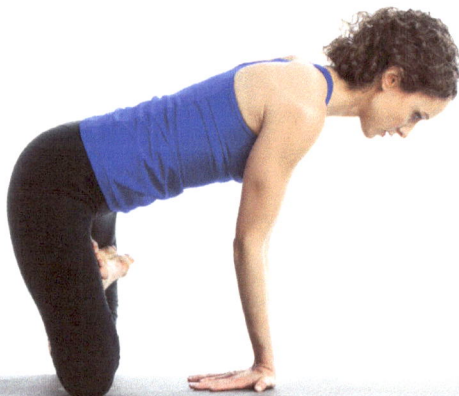

3.2

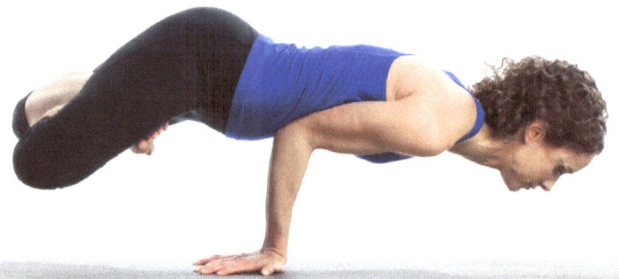

Start from a crossed legged or lotus position and keep your legs in that position for the balance.

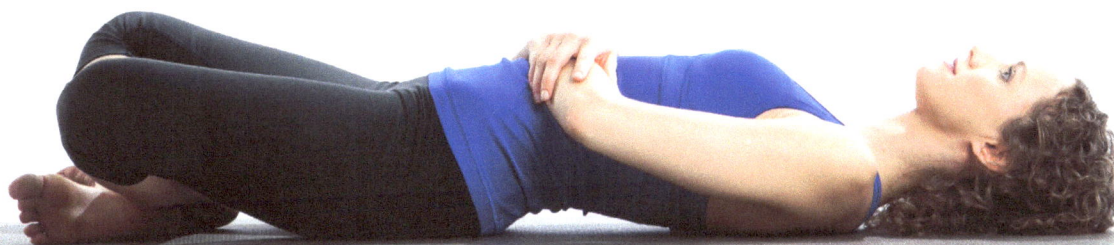

Lie down on your back with your legs crossed and arms resting across your torso.
Inhale.

B

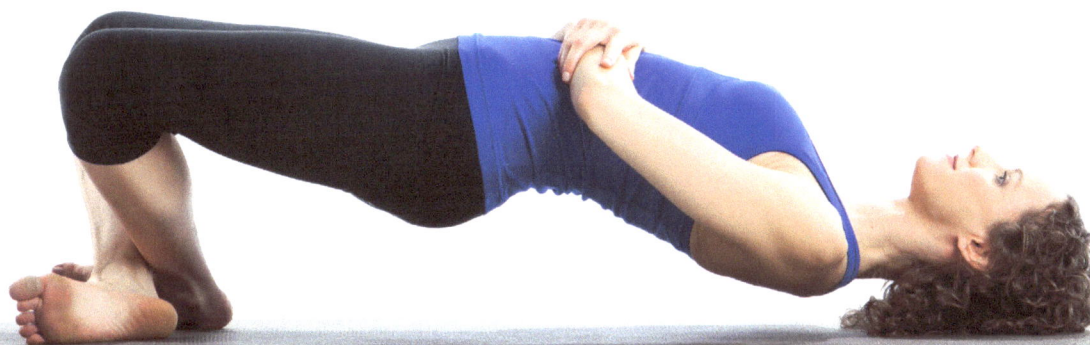

Exhale as you arch your back and press your hips up so that only the pillow spot on the back of your head and feet touch the floor. Tense the back of your neck, glutes, and stomach muscles.

Hold position **B** on each inhalation and tense harder and press higher on each exhalation.

Variations:

I strongly advise starting with variation #1 until you build more strength in the back of your neck.

1.1

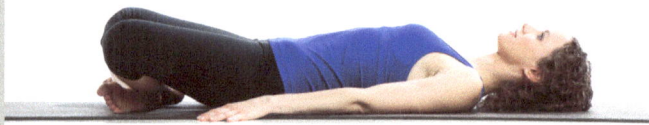

1.2

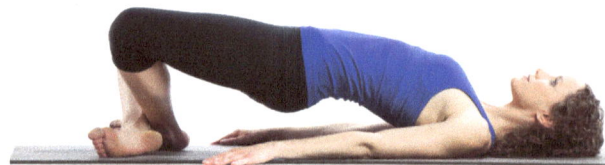

Place your arms on the floor and use your arms to control how much weight you allow on the back of your head.

2.1

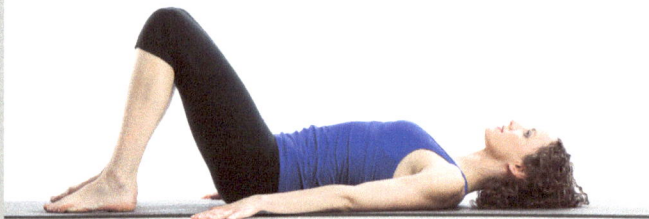

2.2

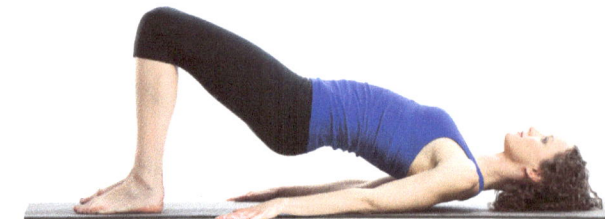

Place your feet next to your hips rather than starting in a crossed legged position.

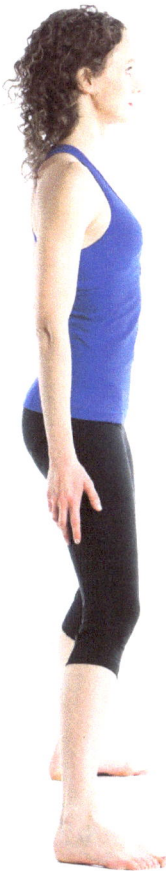

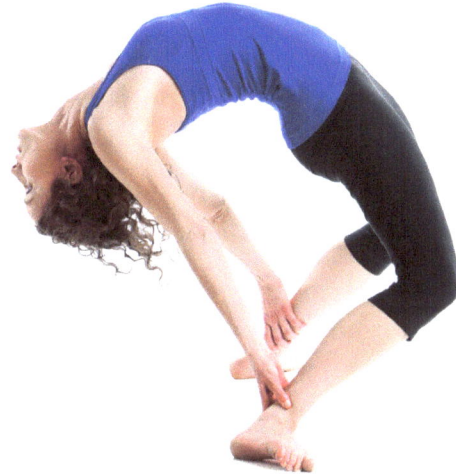

Stand straight with feet in a wide stance and knees bent.
Inhale.

Exhale as you arch back and slowly walk your hands down the backs of your legs until you are touching your ankles. Tense your stomach muscles and glutes.

Hold position **B** on each inhalation and tense harder and bend farther back on each exhalation. Slowly walk your hands back up your legs when you are finished with your repetitions.

Variation:

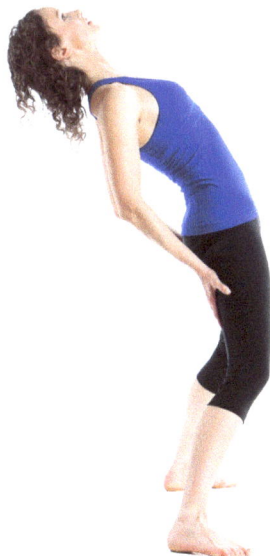

1.1

Start with your hands on your glutes and gradually walk your hands farther down your legs as you build strength and flexibility.

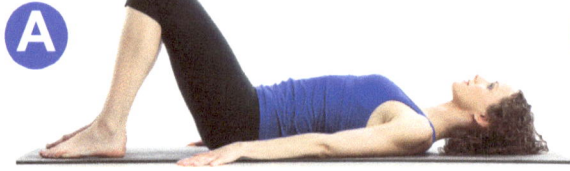

A Lie down on your back with your feet flat and close to your hips.

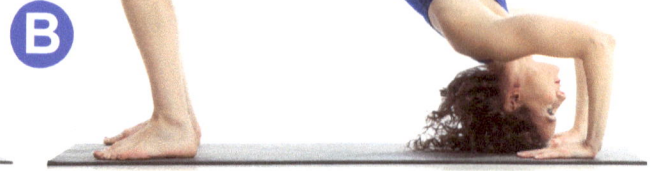

B Place your palms down right above your shoulders and press your hips up so that you can rest the top of your head on the floor.
Inhale.

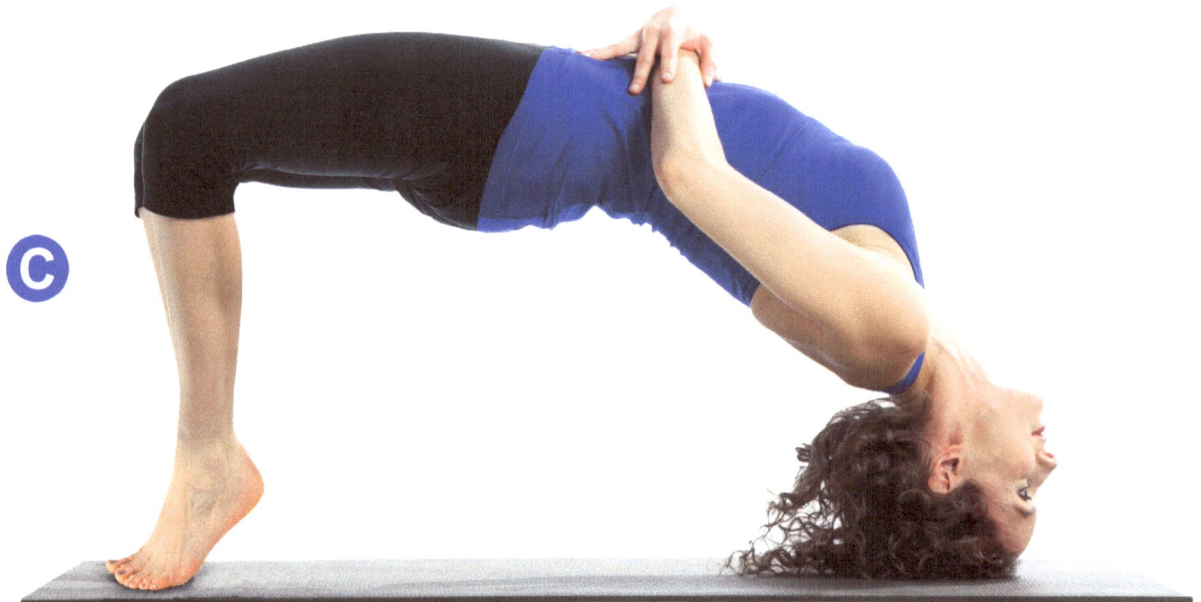

C **Exhale** as you lift your hands off the floor and press up on the balls of your feet. Tense your neck muscles, glutes, and stomach muscles.

Hold position **C** on each inhalation and tense harder and press higher on each exhalation.

Variation:

I strongly advise starting with variation #1 until you build more strength in your neck.

1.1 Keep your hands in place and use your arms to control how much weight you allow on the top of your head.

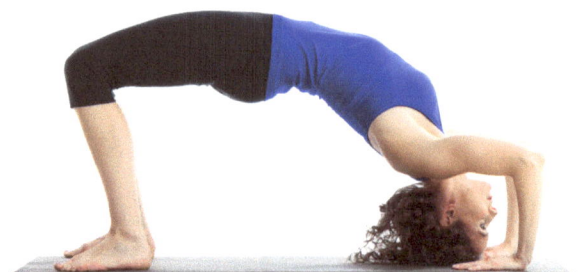

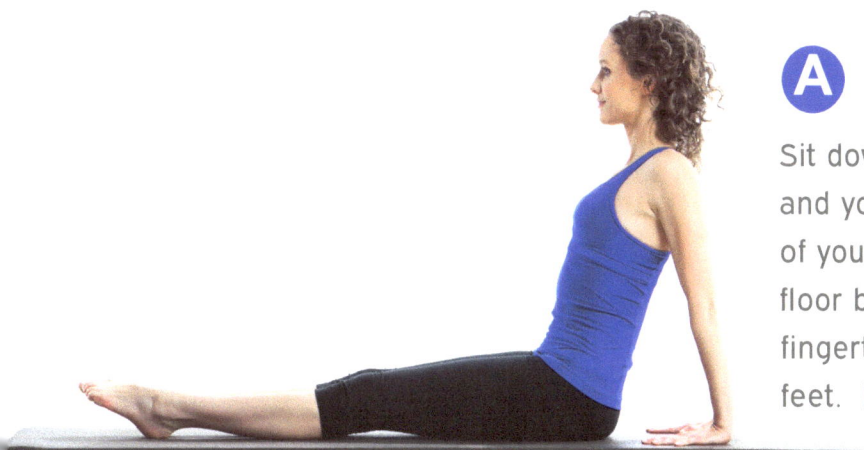

A

Sit down with a straight spine and your legs straight in front of you. Place your palms on the floor behind your hips with your fingertips pointed towards your feet. **Inhale**.

B

Exhale as you press your hips up so that your shoulders, hips, and feet are in a straight line and the bottoms of your feet are touching the floor.

Tense your glutes and hamstrings.

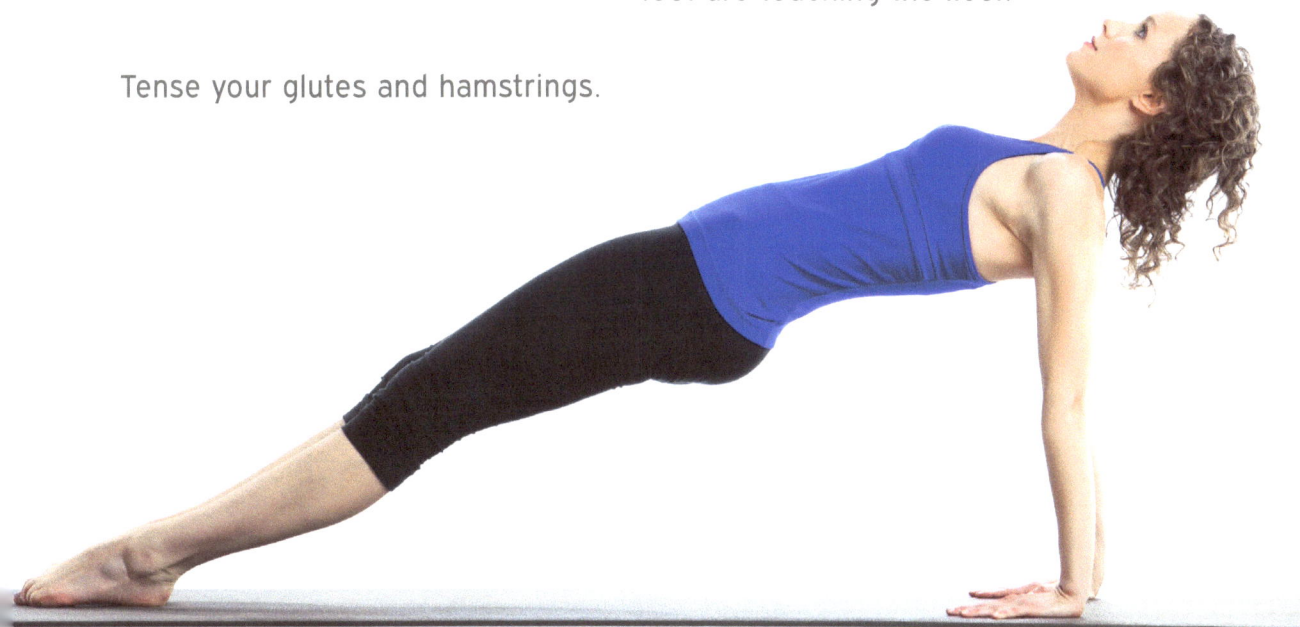

Hold position **B** on each inhalation and tense harder and press higher on each exhalation.

Variation:

1.1

Start with your knees bent and gradually straighten them as you build strength.

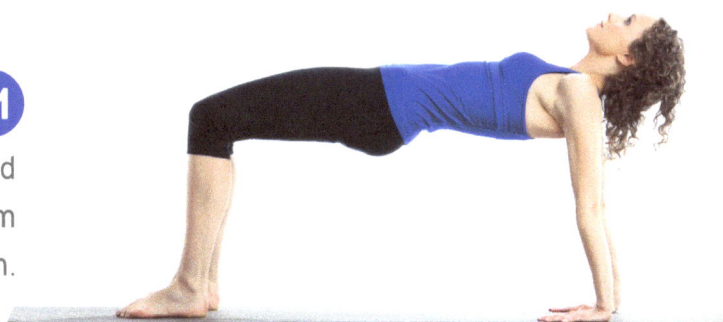

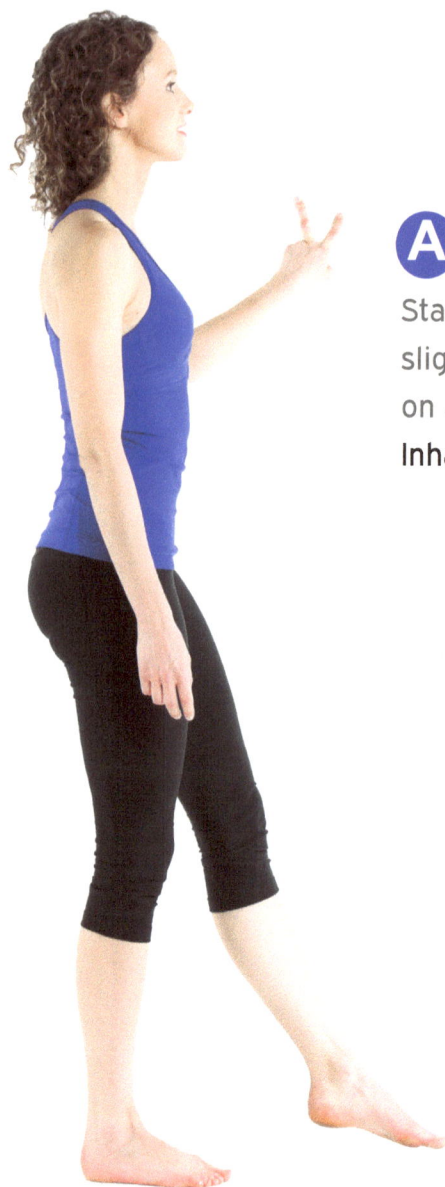

A

Stand straight on one leg with your knee slightly bent. If needed, place two fingers on a wall for balance.
Inhale.

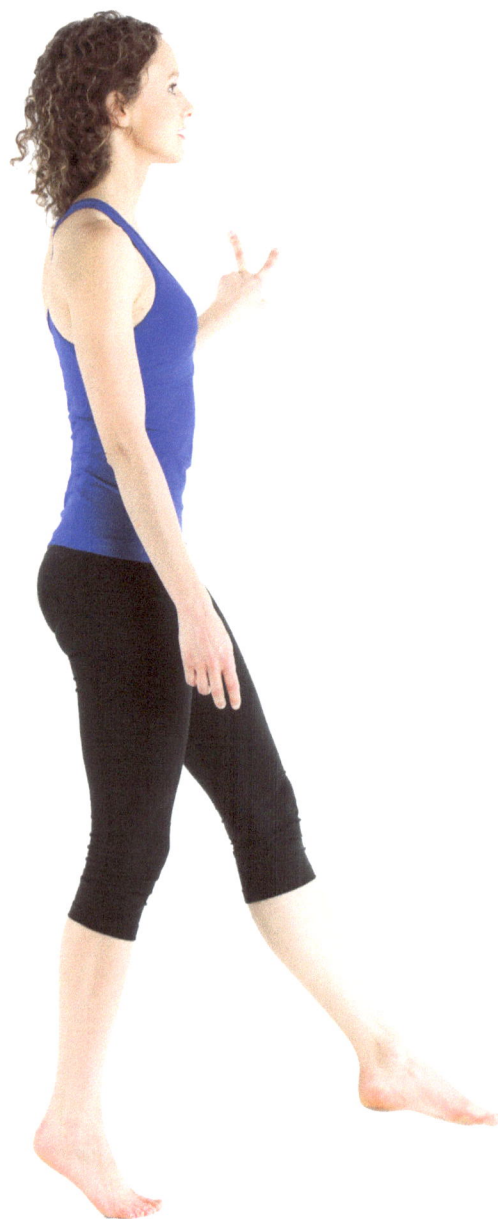

B

Exhale as you push up on the ball of your foot and tense your calf.

Hold position **B** on each inhalation and tense harder on each exhalation. Repeat on the opposite leg for the same number of repetitions.

A

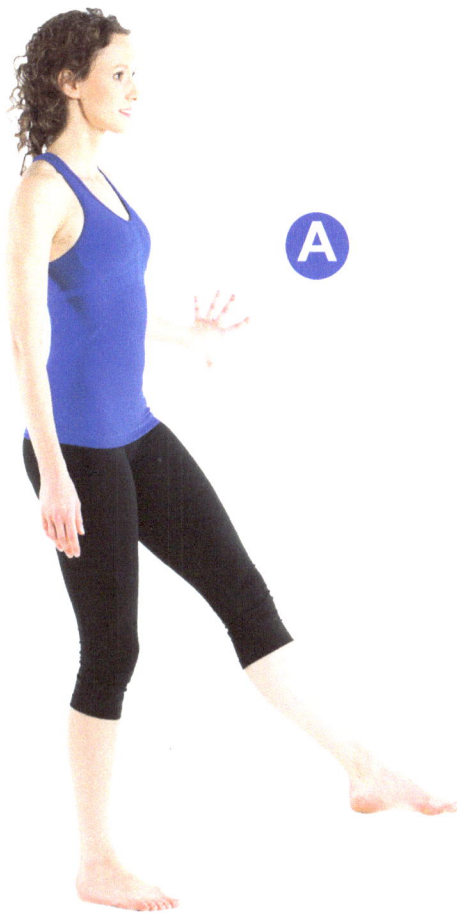

Stand straight on one leg with your knee slightly bent and extend your other leg slightly in front of you.

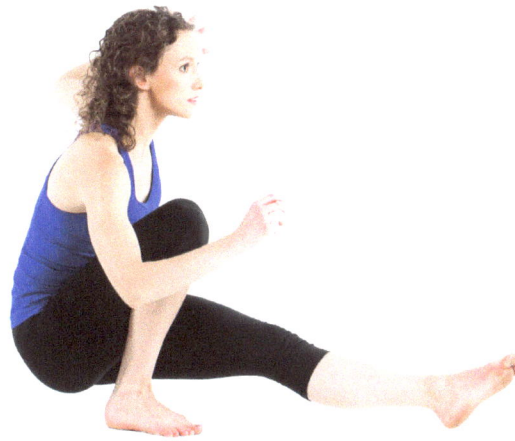

B

Bend your knee, while keeping your foot flat and your hips back, and **inhale** as you lower into a one-legged squat. If needed, place your hand on a wall for balance.

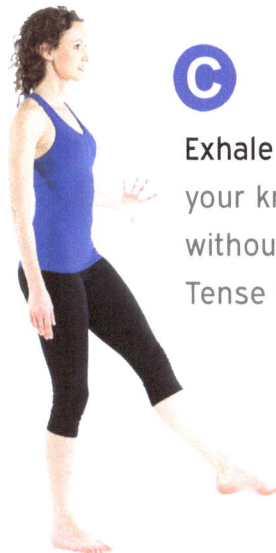

C

Exhale as you straighten your knee back to standing, without locking the knee. Tense your quad.

Lower back down to a one-legged squat on each inhalation and straighten the knee and tense harder on each exhalation. Repeat on the opposite side for the same number of repetitions.

Variation:

1.1

Bend your knee only part of the way into the one-legged squat and gradually bend farther as you build strength.

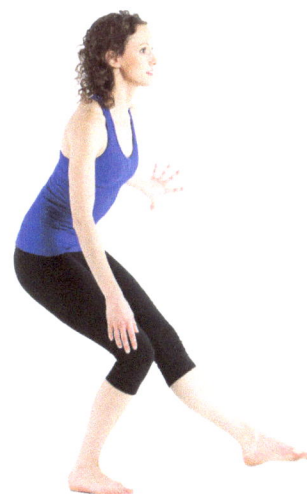

A

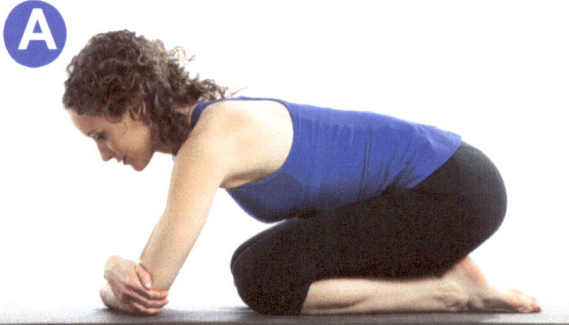

Sit on your feet with your knees close together. Clasp your elbows with your palms and place your elbows on the floor.

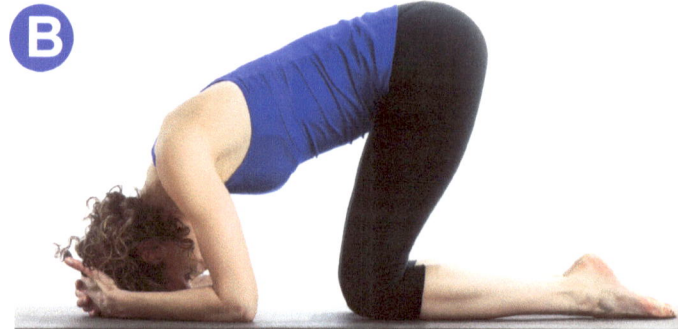

B

Release your elbows and clasp your fingers with your thumbs up. Place the back of your head into your hands.

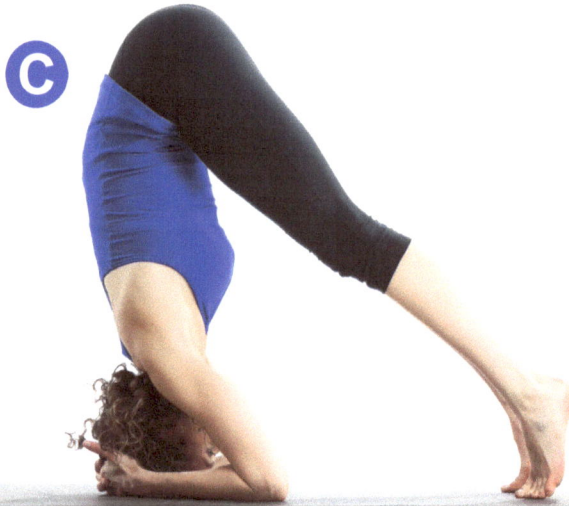

C

Press your hips up and walk your feet towards your face until your hips are above your shoulders.

Be sure that your forearms remain parallel; don't let your elbows spread out to the side.
Inhale.

D

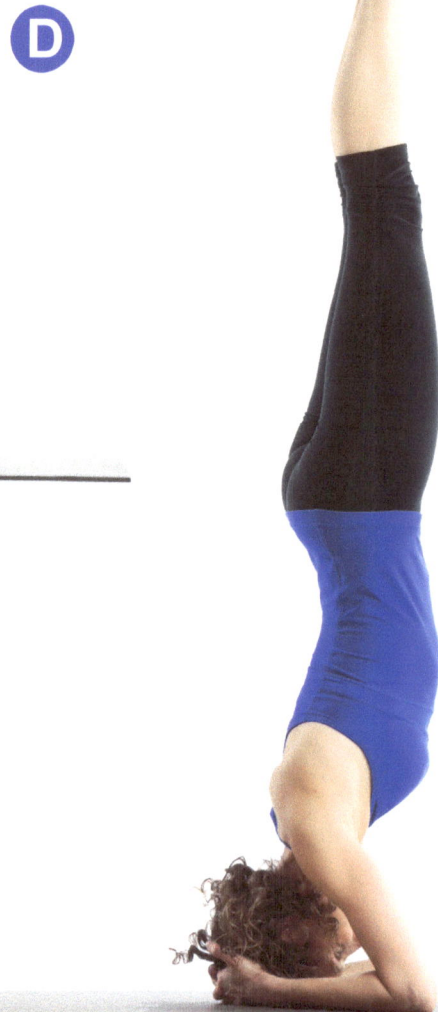

Extend your legs up into a headstand.

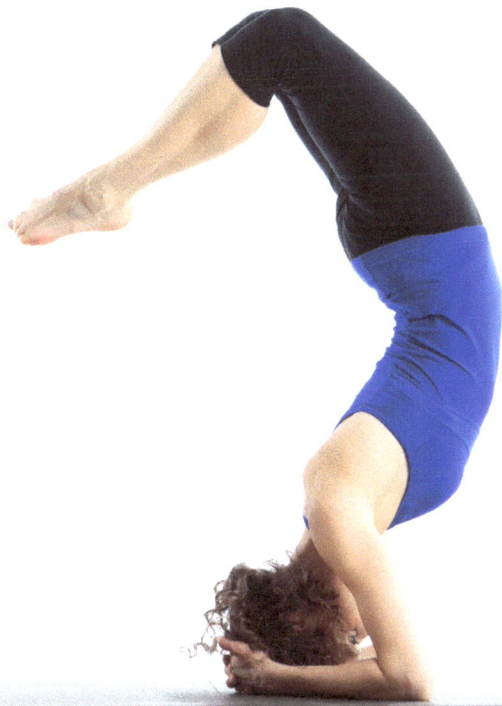

E

Exhale as you arch your back so that your feet are behind you. Tense your stomach muscles, glutes, and back muscles.

2/3 of your body weight should be on your forearms and **1/3** of your body weight is on your head.

Hold position **E** on each inhalation and arch farther and tense harder on each exhalation.

Variations:

1.1

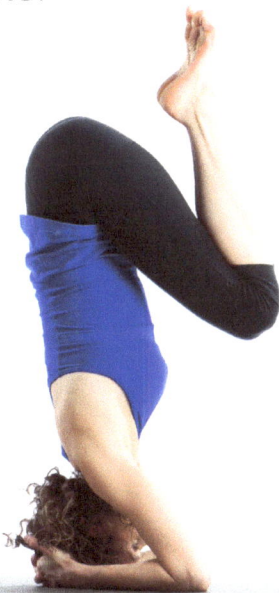

Keep your knees bent and tucked in, then gradually straighten the knees as you build strength. Tense your stomach muscles.

2.1

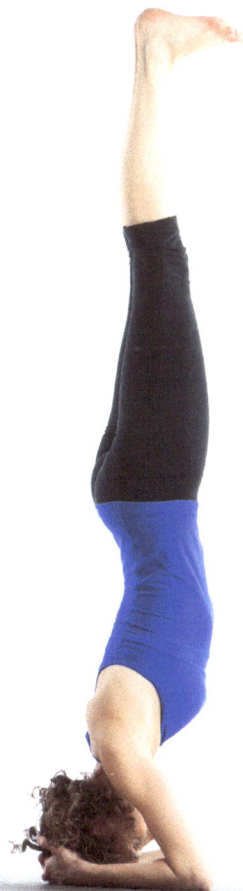

Keep your body completely straight. Tense your entire body.

A

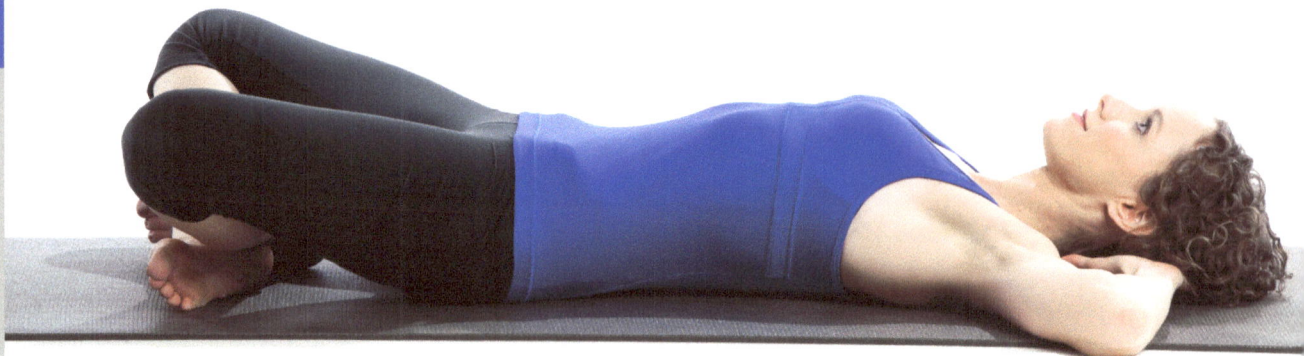

Lie down on your back with your legs crossed.

Touch your fingertips to the back of your head with your elbows out to the side. **Inhale**.

B

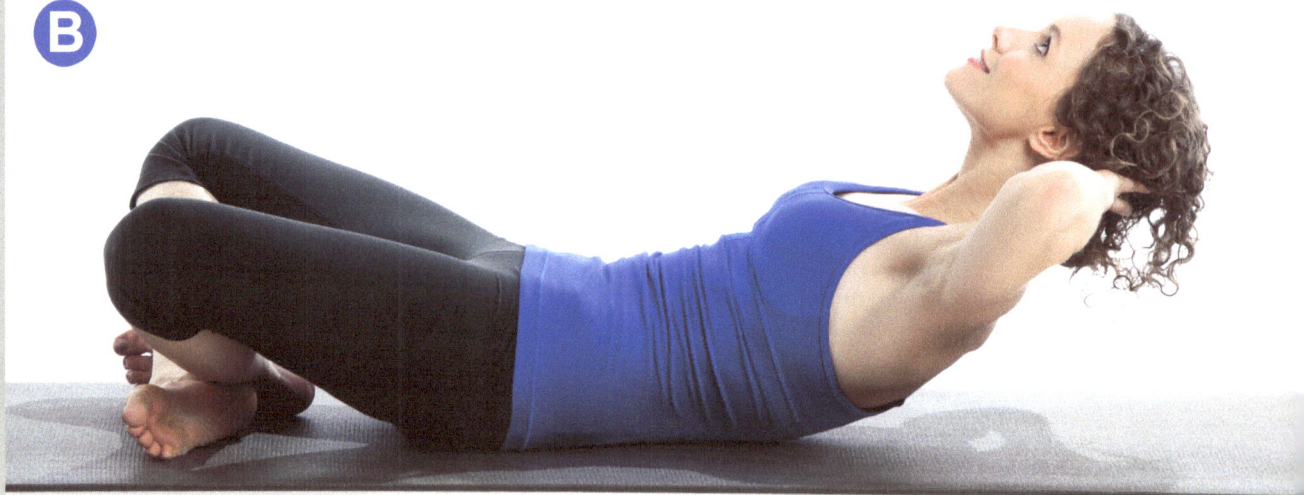

Exhale as you sit up at a 30 degree angle and tense your upper stomach muscles.

Hold position **B** on each inhalation and tense harder on each exhalation.

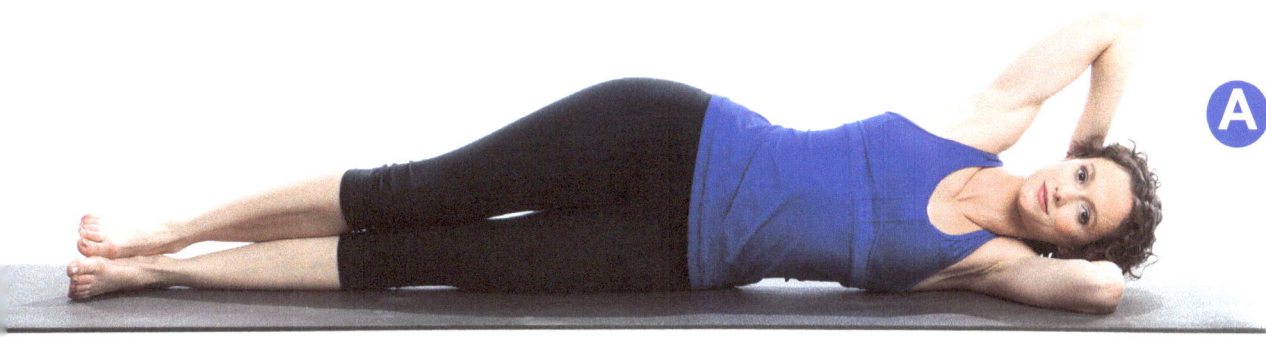

Lie down on your left side with your body straight, so that your shoulders, hips, legs, and feet are stacked on top of each other. Rest your head on your hands.

Inhale.

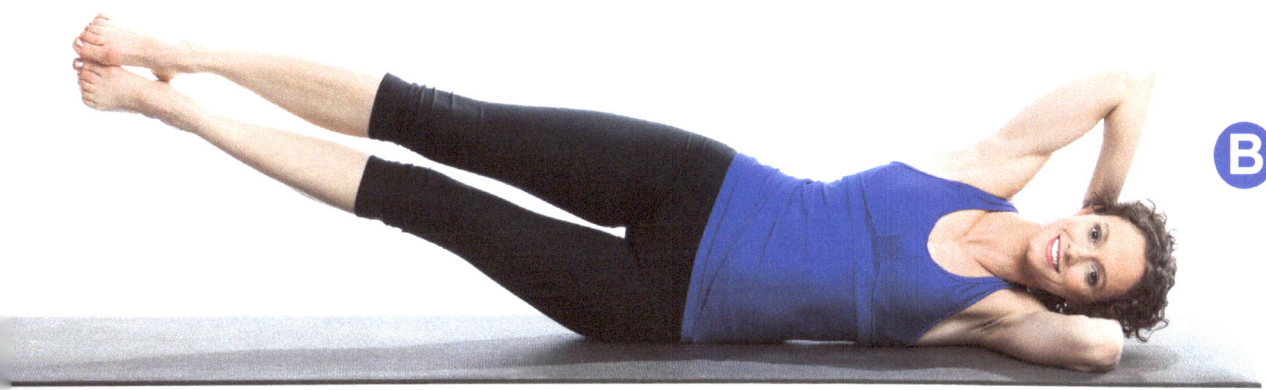

B

Exhale as you lift both legs up and tense your right oblique muscles.

Be sure your body doesn't roll forward or backward as you lift your legs.

Hold position **B** on each inhalation and lift higher and tense harder on each exhalation. Repeat on the opposite side for the same number of repetitions.

Variation:

1.1

Bring your arms in front of your body and press your palms to the floor as you lift your legs.

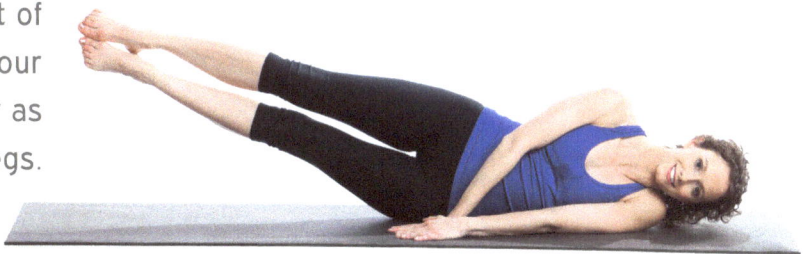

35

A

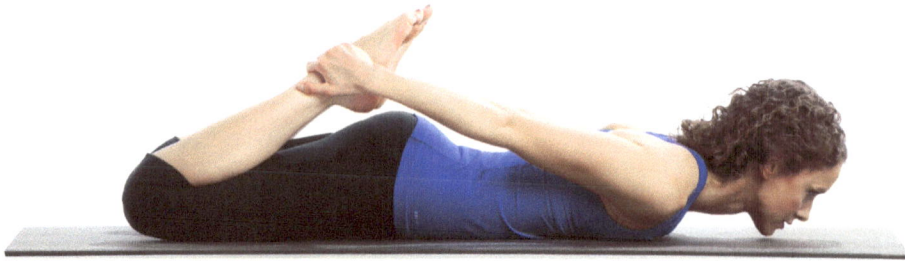

Lie face down and bend your knees so you can grab your ankles.
Your knees should be shoulder width apart.
Inhale.

B

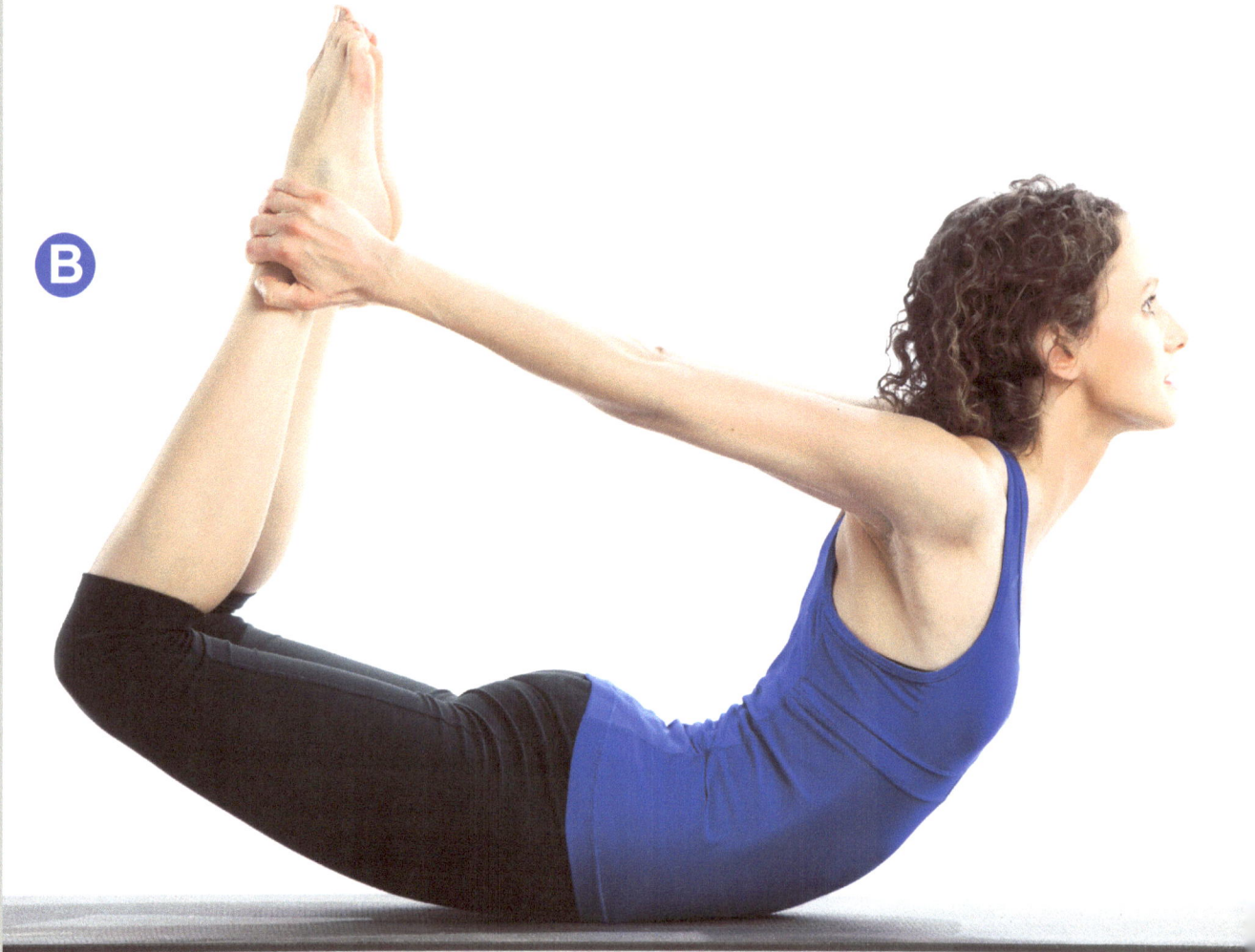

Exhale as you try to straighten your legs so that your chest will lift off the floor for a stomach stretch.

Hold position **B** on each inhalation and stretch farther on each exhalation.

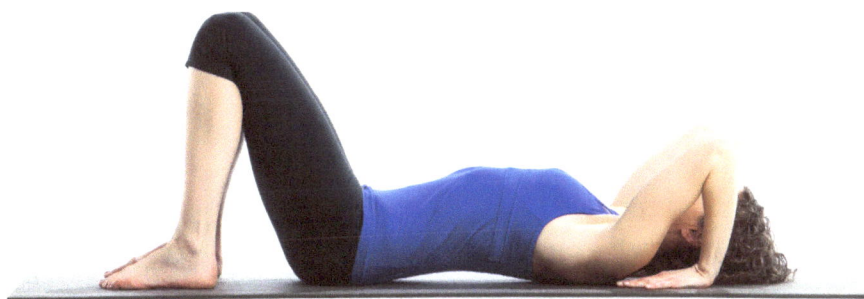

Lie down on your back with your feet flat and close to your hips. Place your palms on the floor right above your shoulders with your fingers pointing towards your body. **Inhale**.

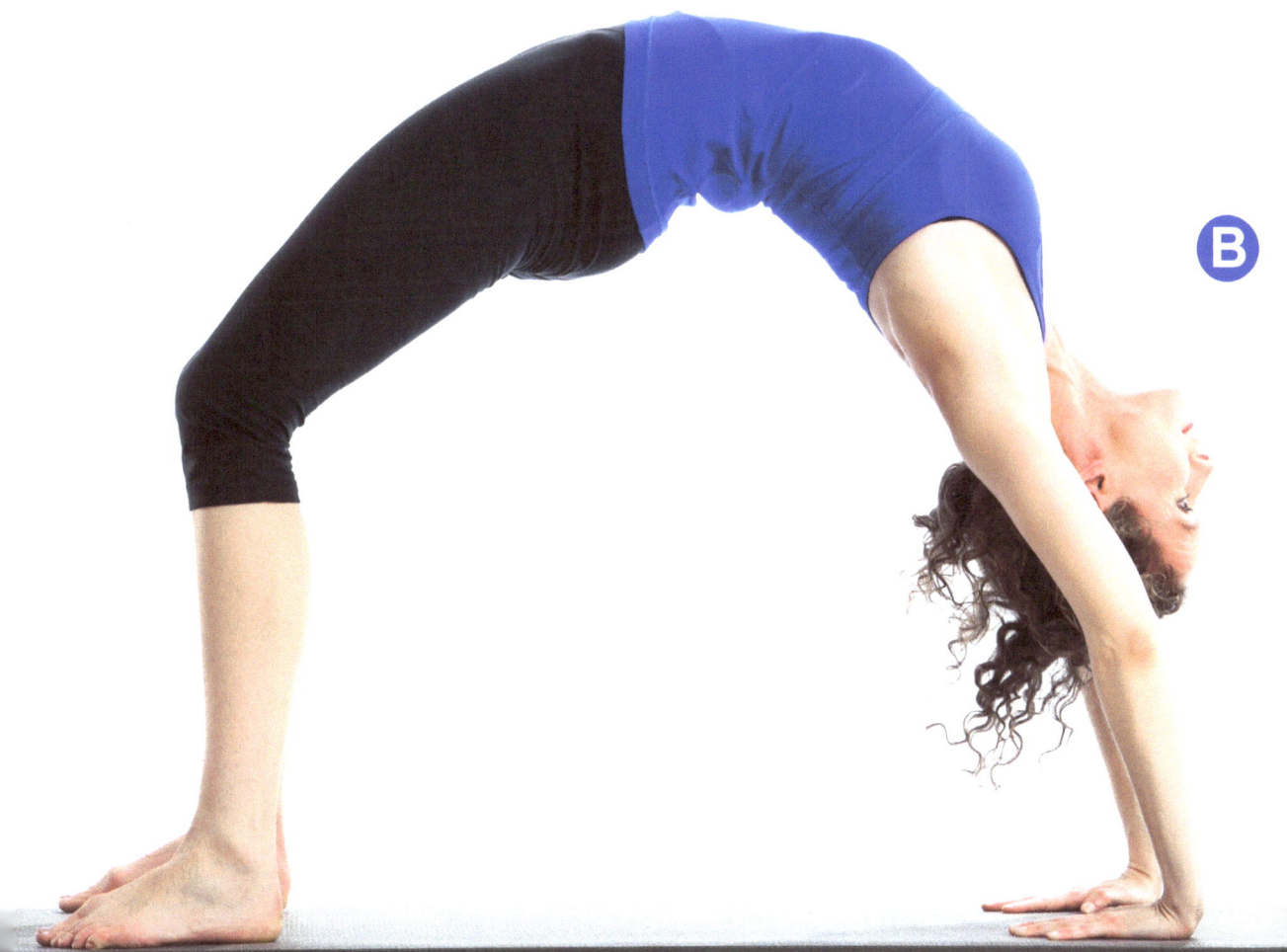

B

Exhale as you press your hips up and arch your back so only your feet and palms touch the floor for a stomach stretch. Tense your glutes and stomach muscles.

Hold position **B** on each inhalation and tense harder and press your hips higher on each exhalation.

37

A

B

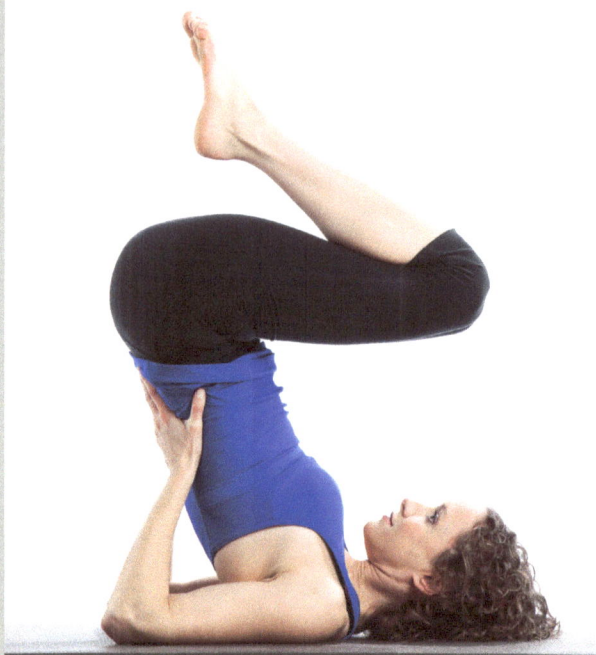

Lie down on your back and lift your legs up so that your weight is on your shoulders, not your neck or head.

Support your lower back with your hands.
Inhale.

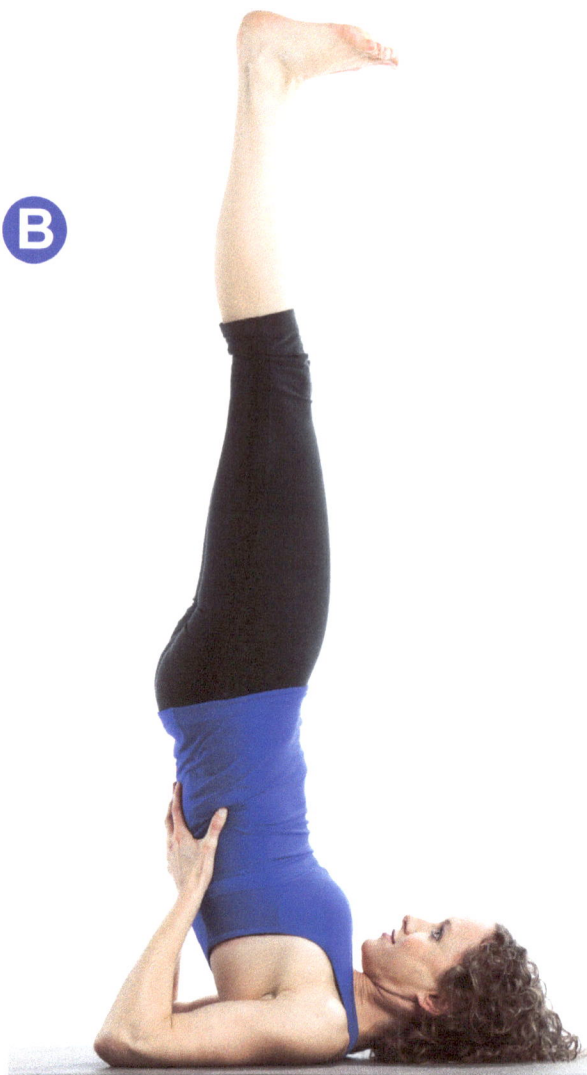

Exhale as your straighten your body and legs and flex your feet so your heels press towards the ceiling.

Tense your entire body.

Hold position **B** on each inhalation and tense harder and press higher on each exhalation.

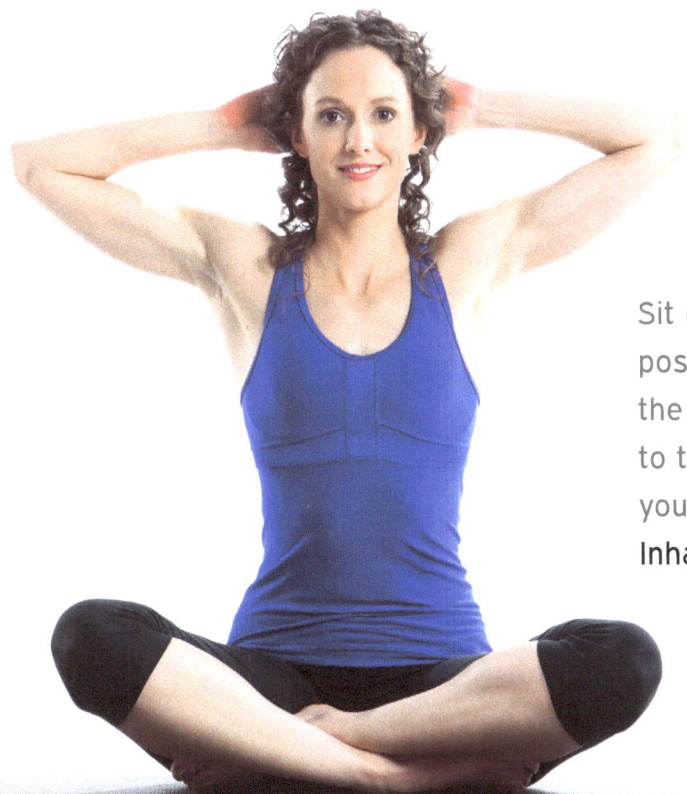

Sit down in a crossed legged position with your right leg on the outside. Touch your fingertips to the back of your head with your elbows out to the side. **Inhale**.

B

Exhale as you twist your right elbow to your left knee for a spinal twist stretch.

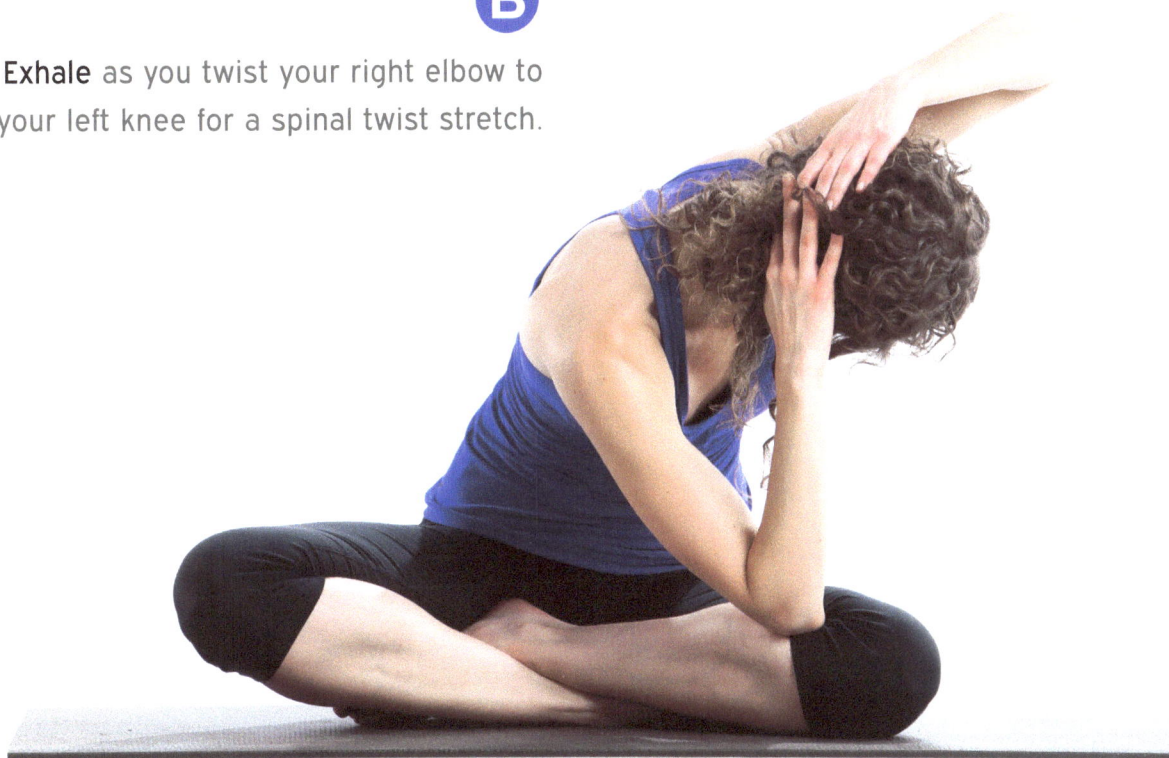

Hold position B on each inhalation and stretch farther on each exhalation. Repeat on the opposite side for the same number of repetitions.

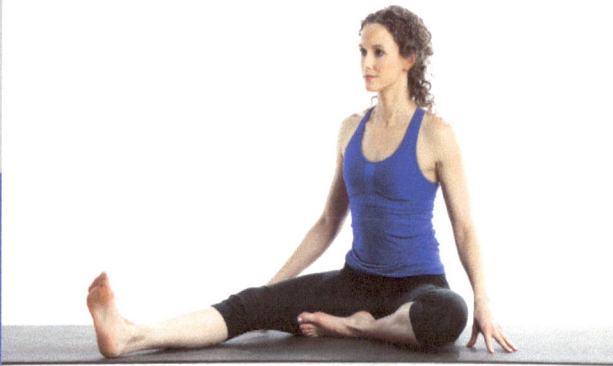

A

Sit down with a straight spine and extend your right leg directly in front of you. Place your left foot into your right inner thigh, as high up as possible. **Inhale.**

B

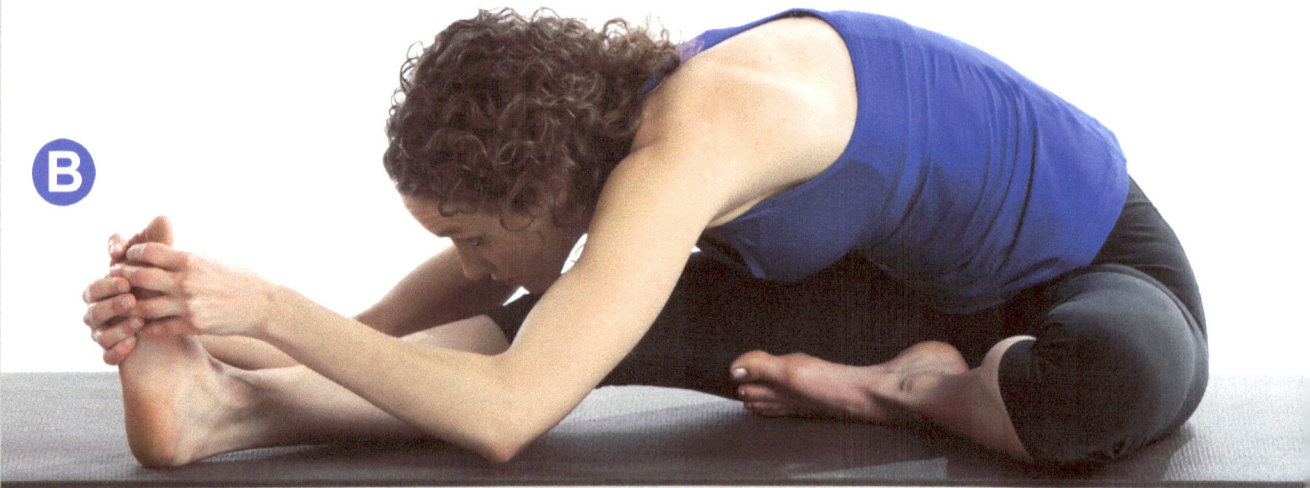

Exhale as you bend forward with a straight spine and clasp the ball of your right foot with both hands for a hamstring stretch.
Attempt to touch your forehead or eventually your chin to your knee and keep your right foot flexed, while maintaining a relatively straight spine.

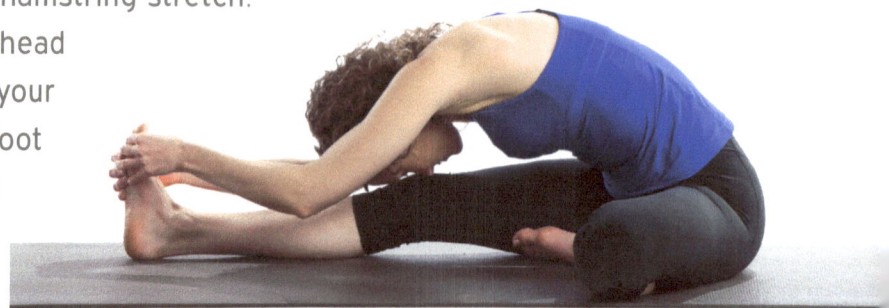

Hold position **B** on each inhalation and stretch farther on each exhalation. Repeat on the opposite side for the same number of repetitions.

Variation:

Most of the variations in this book make the exercise easier. This one is harder!

1.1

Place the top of your left foot across your right thigh for an added left hip stretch.

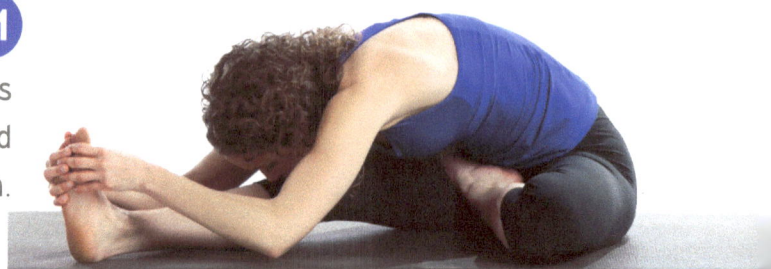

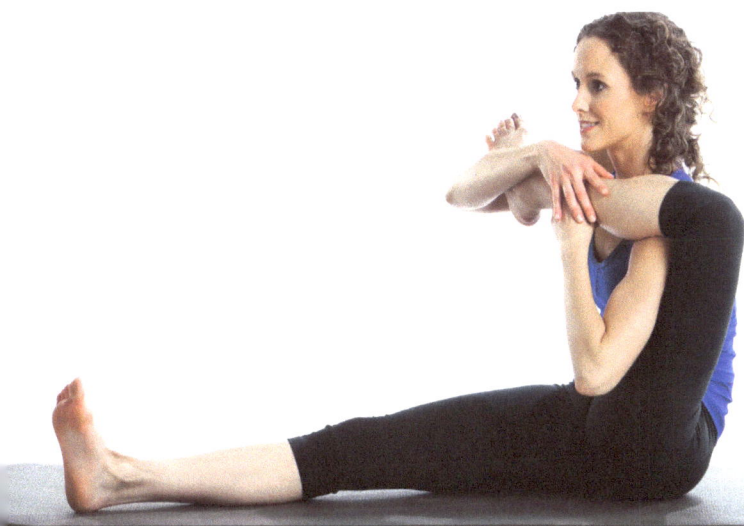

A

Sit down with a straight spine and extend your right leg directly in front of you.

Bring your left knee up over your left shoulder and pull your left foot towards your right shoulder.
Inhale.

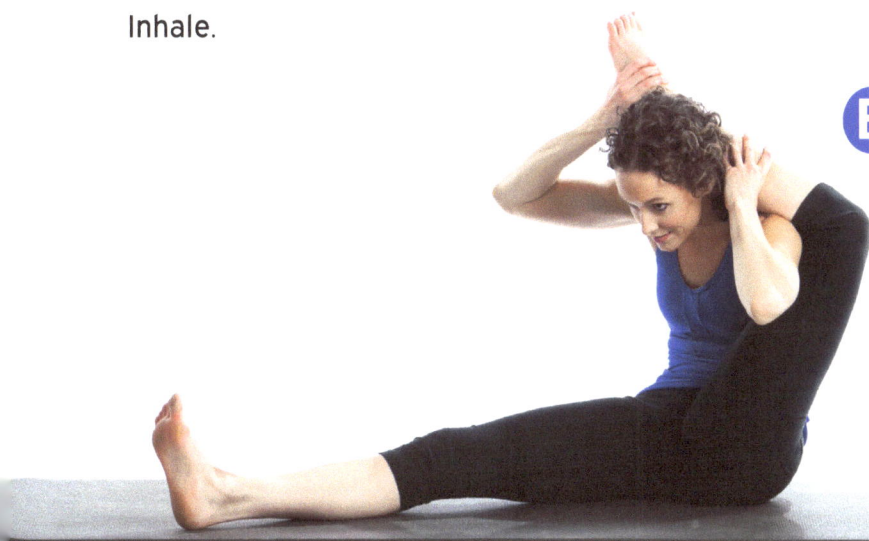

B

Exhale as you pull your left foot up and behind your head for a hip stretch.

C

Once you can easily get your foot behind your head, bend forward with a straight spine and clasp the ball of your right foot with your right hand.

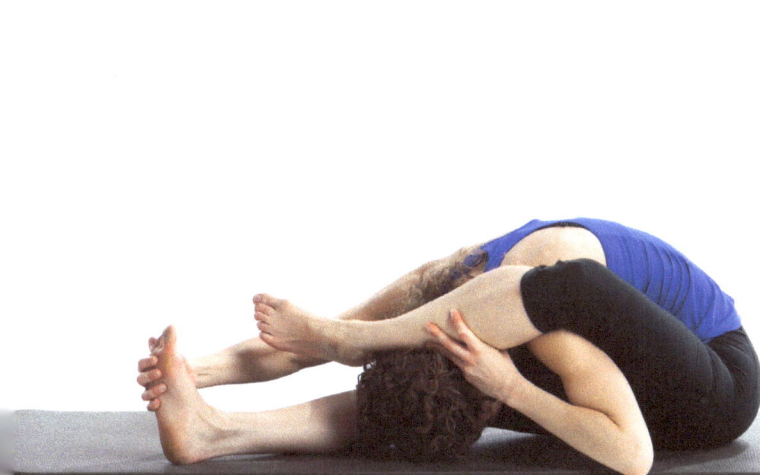

Hold position **B**, or eventually position **C**, on each inhalation and stretch farther on each exhalation. Repeat on the opposite side for the same number of repetitions.

Variations:

1.1

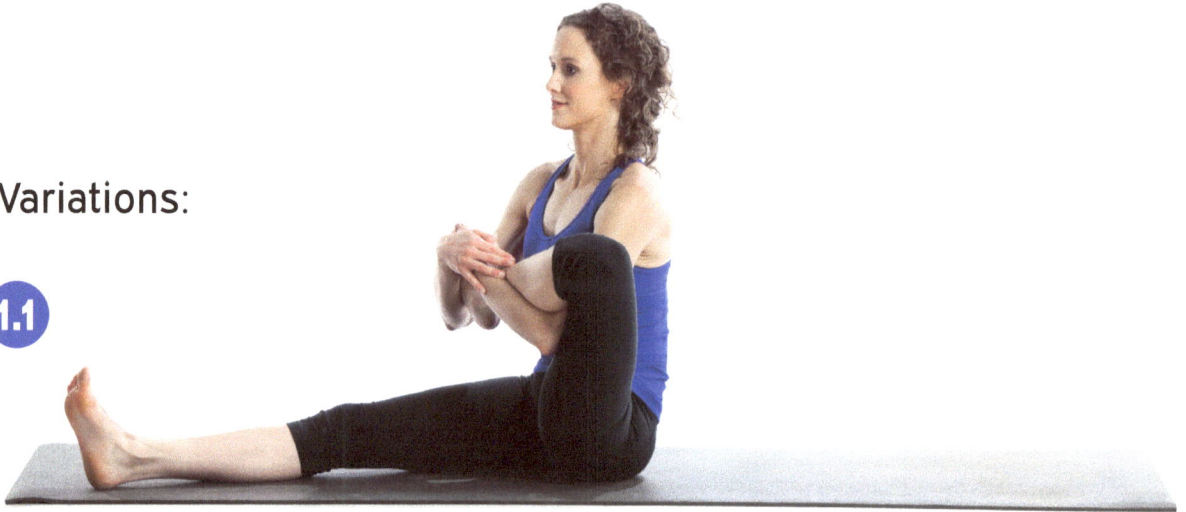

Hook your left elbow under your left knee and pull your left foot to your right elbow.

1.2

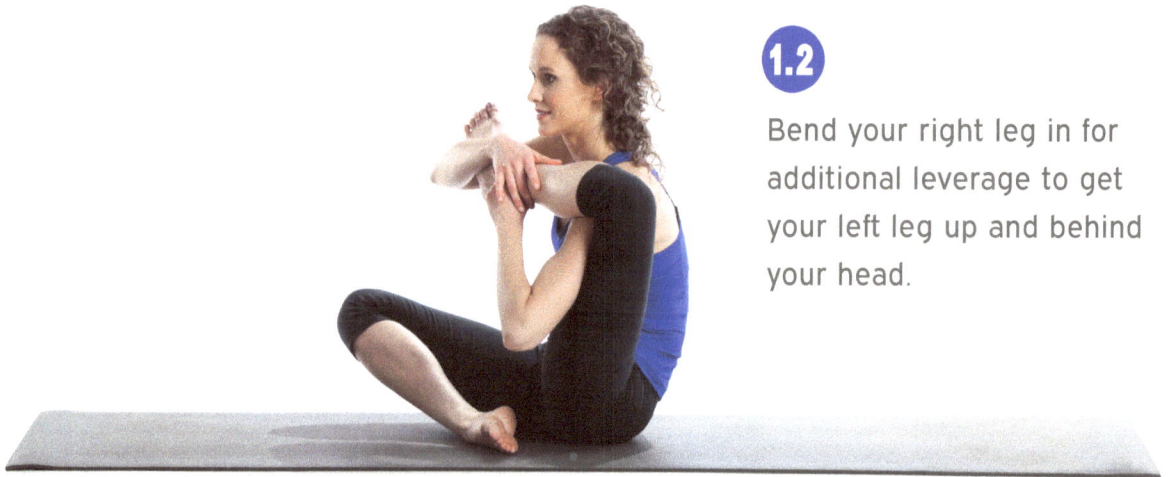

Bend your right leg in for additional leverage to get your left leg up and behind your head.

1.3

Lean back once your foot is behind your head, either with a straight or bent right leg.

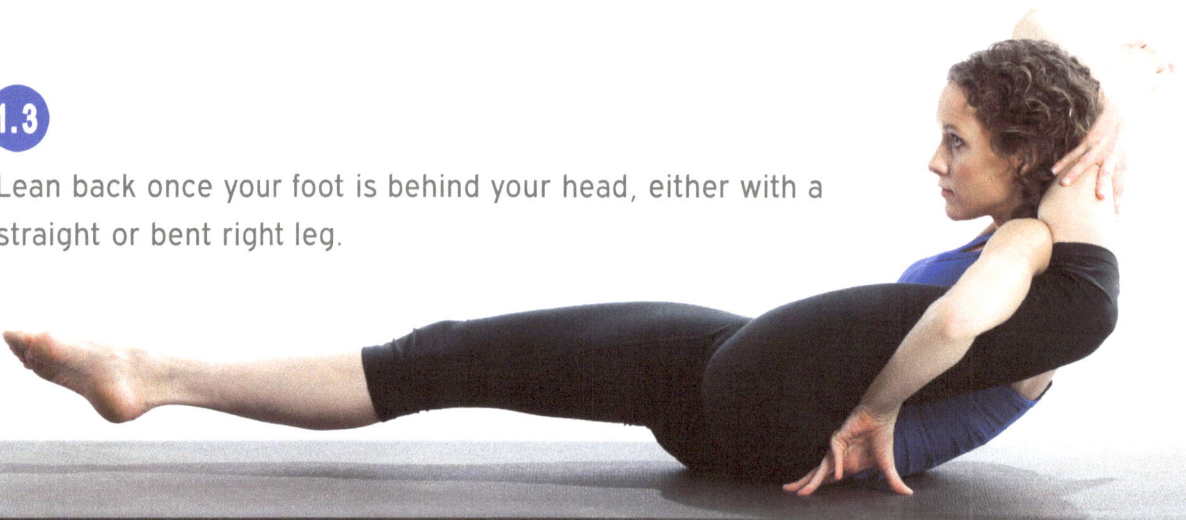

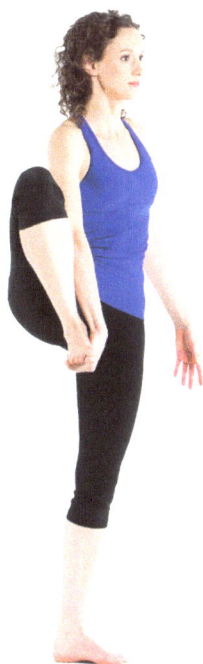 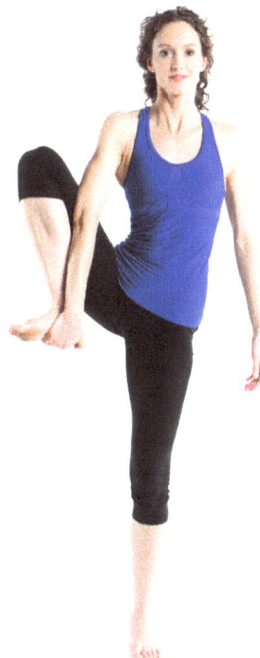

Stand straight on your left leg with your knee slightly bent. Clasp the inside of your right foot with your right hand. If needed, place two fingers on a wall for balance.

Inhale.

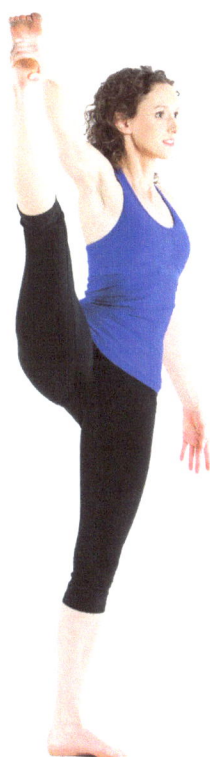 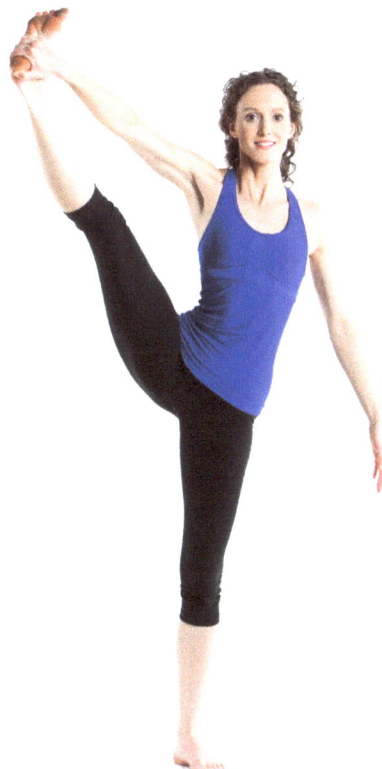

B

Exhale as you extend the right leg as far out and as high as you can for a hamstring stretch.

Hold position **B** on each inhalation and stretch farther on each exhalation. Repeat on the opposite side for the same number of repetitions.

42

A

Squat down on the balls of your feet with your heels almost touching and your toes pointed to the sides. Place your palms down in front of your feet with your fingertips pointed forward. **Inhale**.

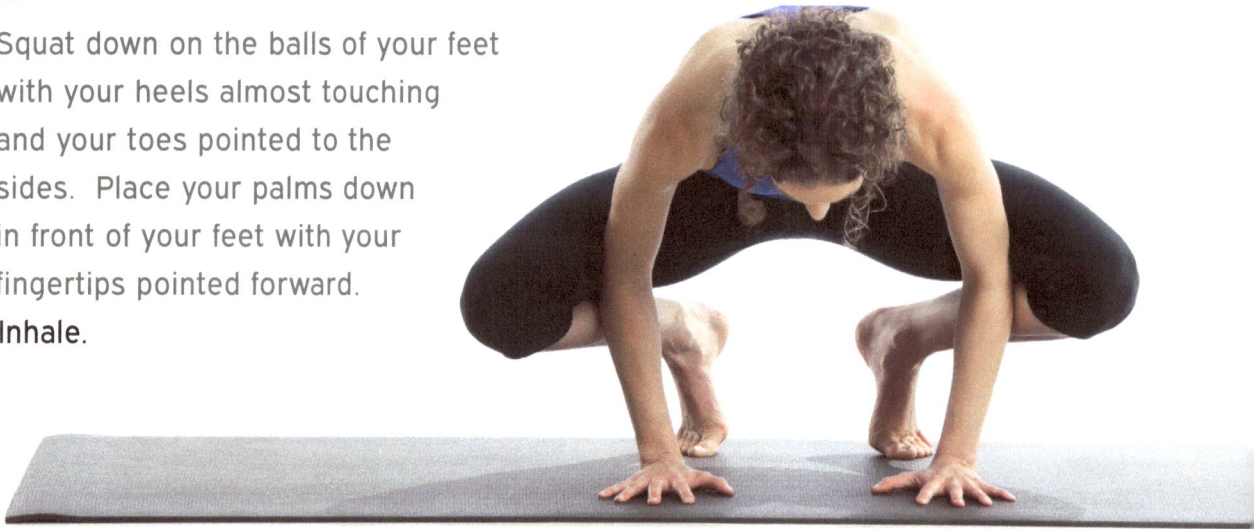

B

Exhale as you place your inner thighs on your elbows and slowly bring your weight forward to balance on your hands for an inner thigh stretch and balance exercise.

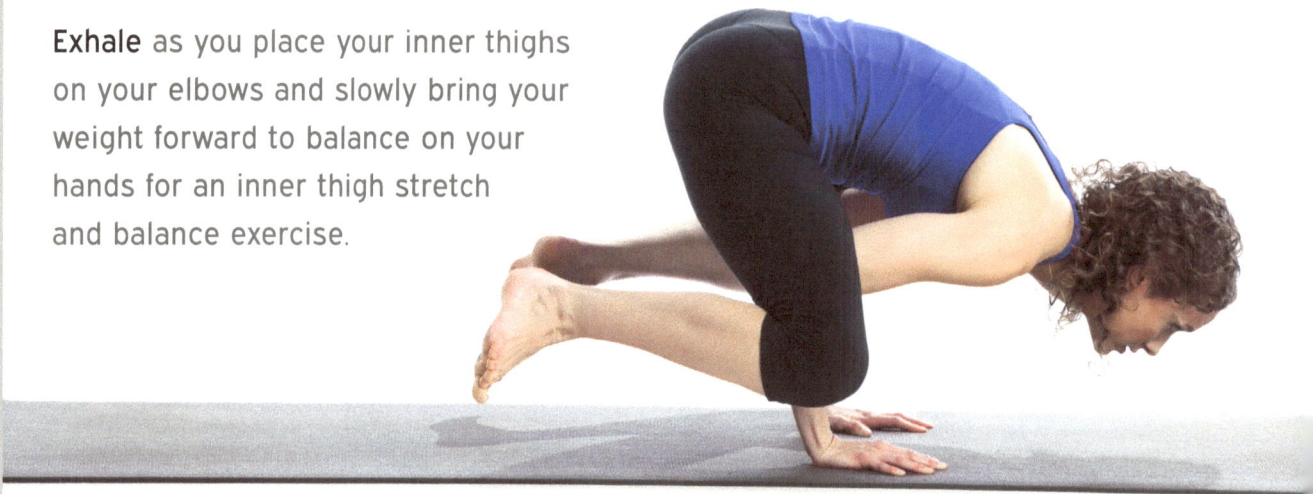

Tense your glutes and stomach muscles and look forward instead of at your feet to help keep your balance.

Hold position **B** on each inhalation and press your knees out wider on each exhalation.

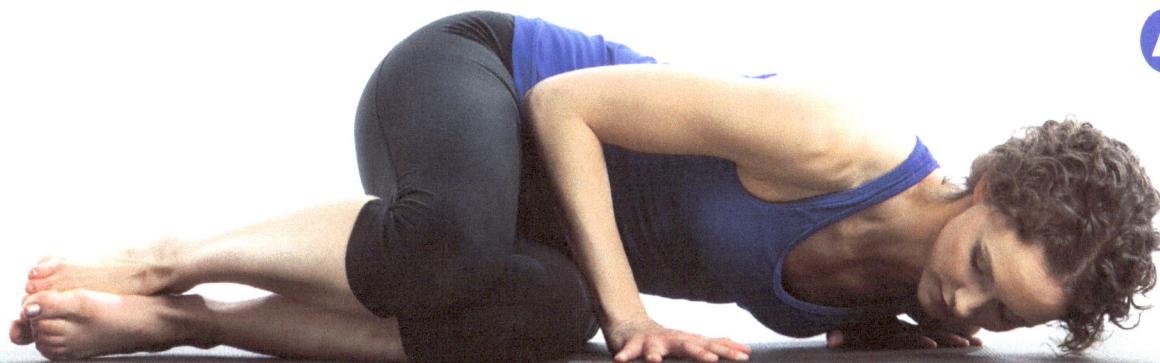

Lie down on your left side with your knees bent and tucked close to your body.

Place palms on the floor in front of your chest and stomach. **Inhale.**

B

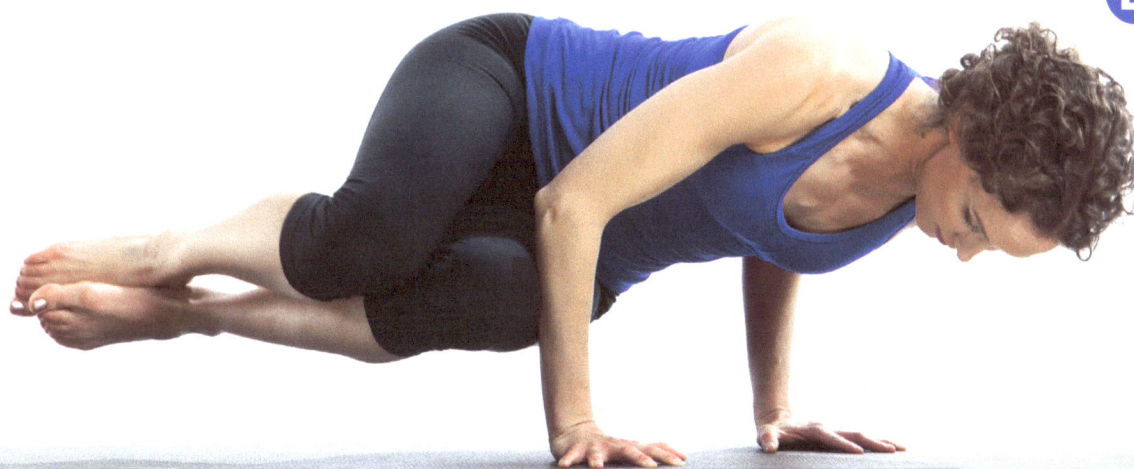

Exhale as your press your body, including your legs, off the floor so that only your hands are touching the floor.

Tense your entire body, particularly your right glutes and oblique muscles and both arms.

Hold position B on each inhalation and tense harder and press higher on each exhalation. Repeat on the opposite side for the same number of repetitions.

Variations:

*This was the toughest exercise for me to get and I can still only hold position **B** for a moment before I crash to the floor. Don't get discouraged if you have difficulty with #43. All of the variations here work different aspects of the exercise, so I recommend practicing all the variations regularly.*

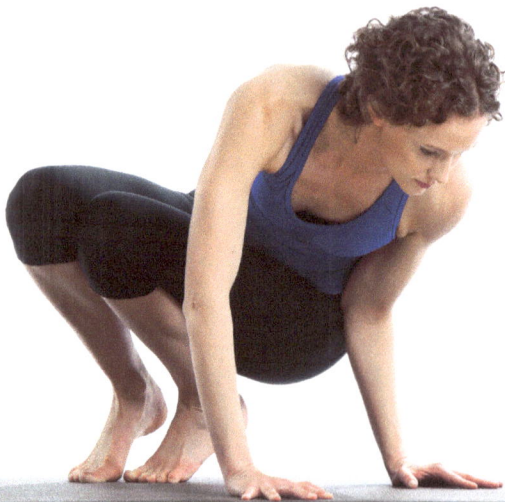

1.1

Squat down on the balls of your feet and twist your knees to the right.

Place your left hip/side into your left elbow to help hold your body off the floor.

1.2

Lean forward and pick your weight up off the floor.

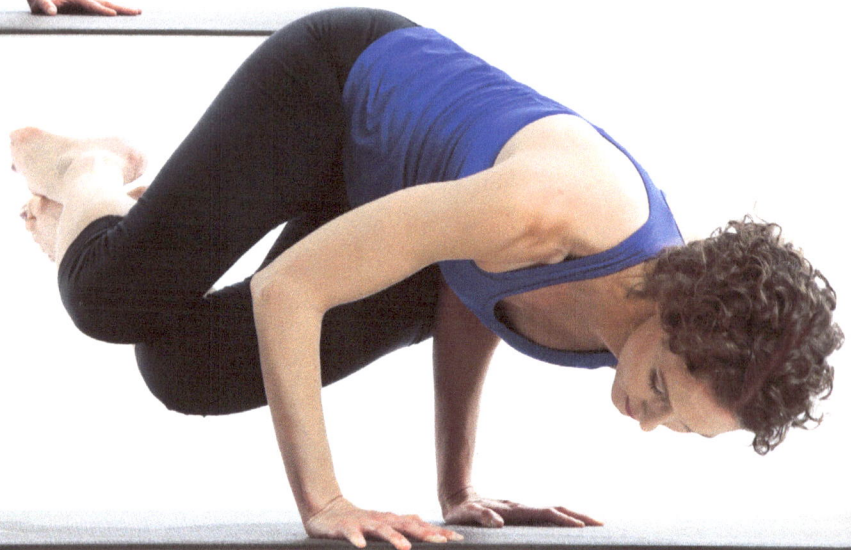

2.1

Squat down on the balls of your feet and twist your knees to the right.

Place your left outer thigh on your right elbow.

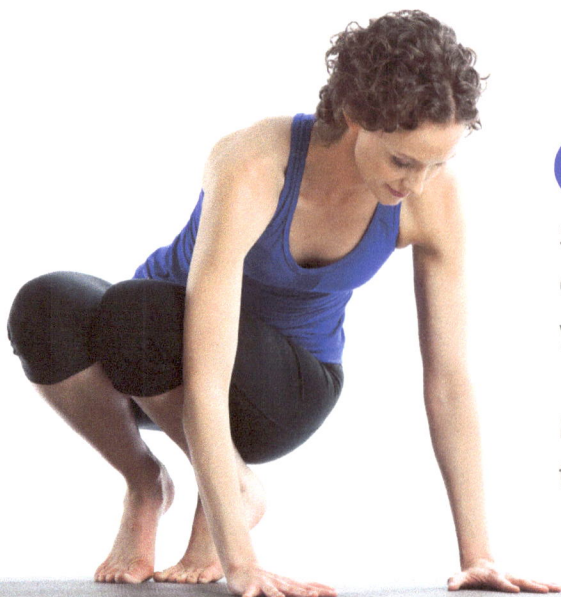

2.2

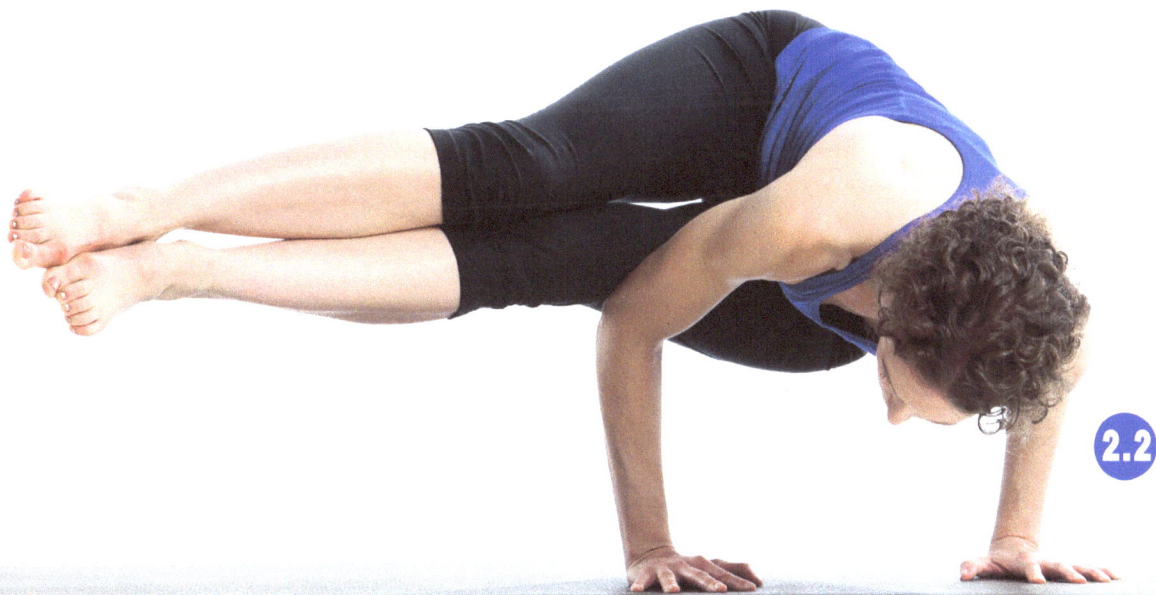

Lean forward and pick your weight up off the floor by releasing your left foot off the floor, then your right. Stack your knees on top of each other.

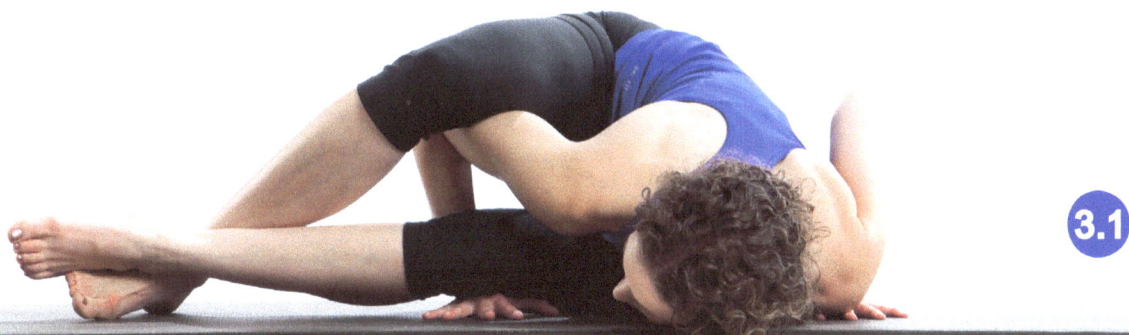

3.1

Lie down on your left side with your knees bent and tucked close to your body. Place your left palm down near your left shoulder.

Weave your right arm between your knees and place your right palm down at your knees.

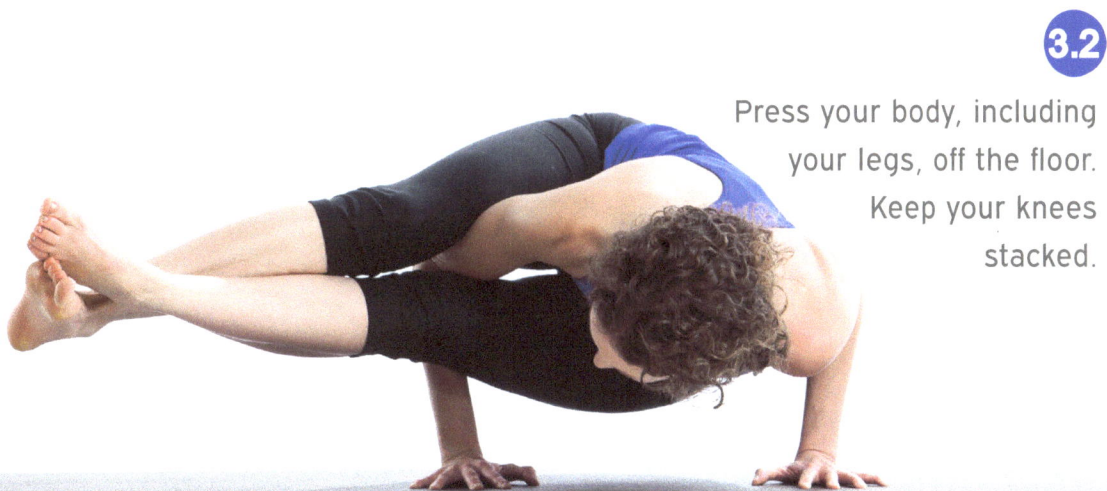

3.2

Press your body, including your legs, off the floor. Keep your knees stacked.

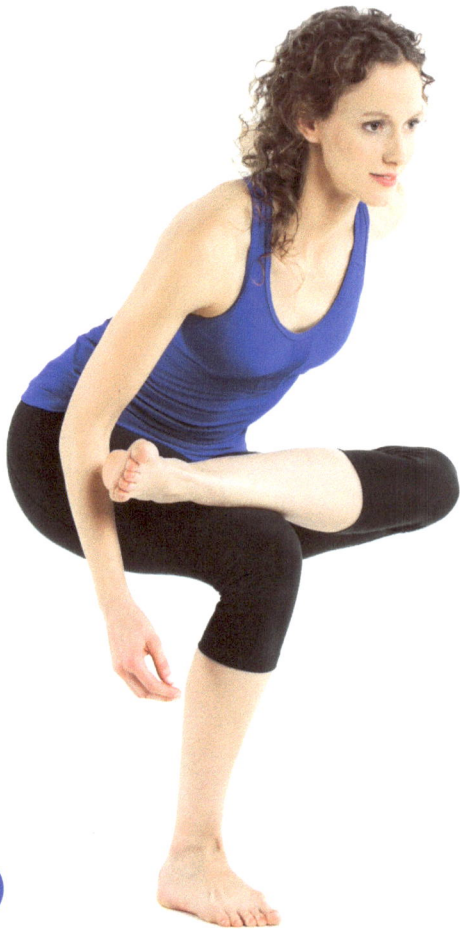

A

Squat down on your right leg with your left ankle crossed above your right knee.

If needed, place two fingers on a wall for balance.
Inhale.

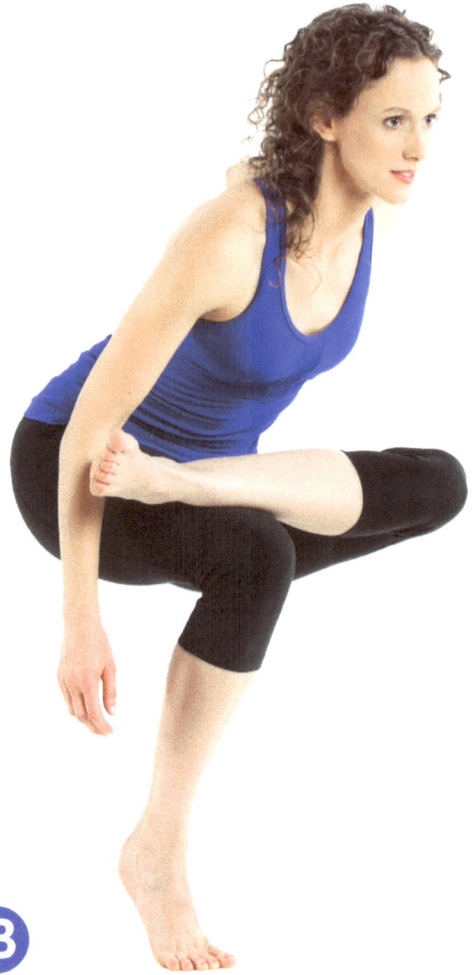

B

Lift your right heel slightly off the floor.

Exhale as you press your heel higher off the floor for a calf raise. Tense your calf muscle.

Lower your heel down on each inhalation and tense harder and press higher on each exhalation.

Repeat on the opposite side for the same number of repetitions.

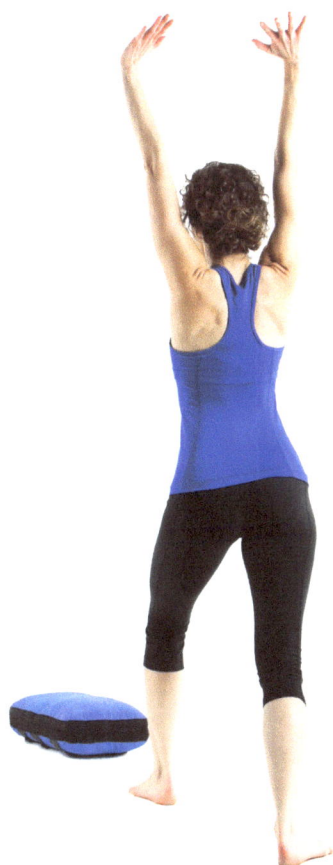

A

Stand in a shallow lunge with your left foot forward, facing a wall with your hands above your head.

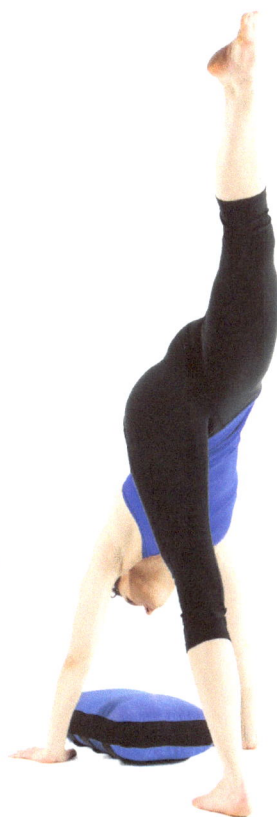

B

Bend forward with a straight spine while you lift your right leg until your palms touch the floor.

Always place a cushion underneath your head before you kick up to your handstand to protect your head and neck in case your arm muscles tire out.

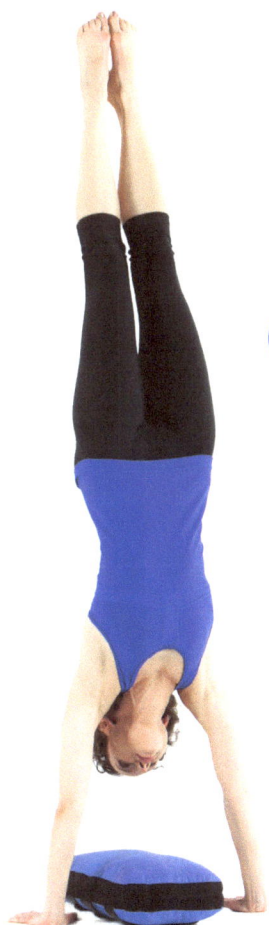

C

Kick off the left leg and bring both legs above your head to a handstand on the wall.

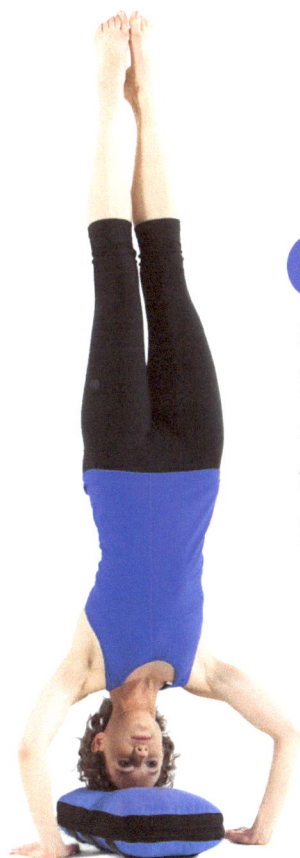

D

Inhale as you lower half way down to the floor for a handstand pushup.

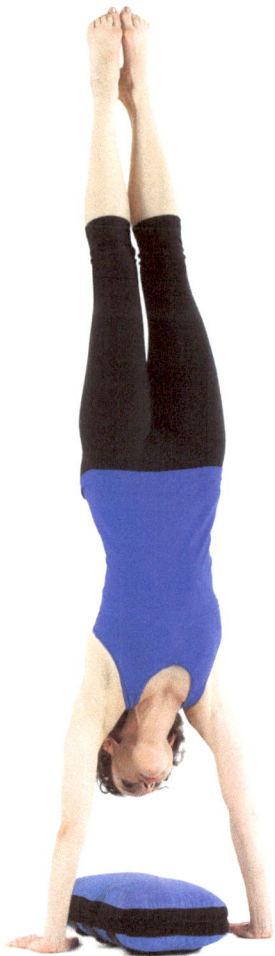

E

Exhale as you press back up to a handstand by straightening your arms. Tense both arms, shoulders, upper back, glutes, and stomach muscles. Be sure to keep your body straight; don't let your lower back arch.

Lower half way back down to a handstand pushup on each inhalation and straighten your arms and tense harder on each exhalation.

Variations:

1.1

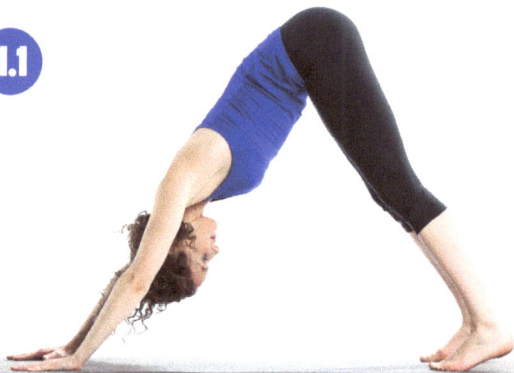

Place your palms and feet on the floor and press your hips to the ceiling so that your body is in a V shape.

Your hands, shoulders, and hips should be in a straight line and your lower back should be flat.

1.2

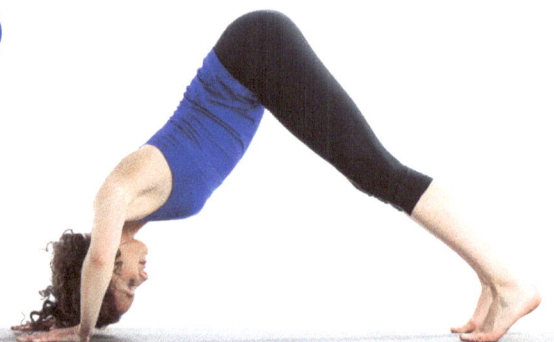

Look at your belly button and lower the top of your head to the floor on each inhalation and straighten your arms on each exhalation for a shoulder pushup.

Tense both arms and shoulders and your upper back during the exhalation.

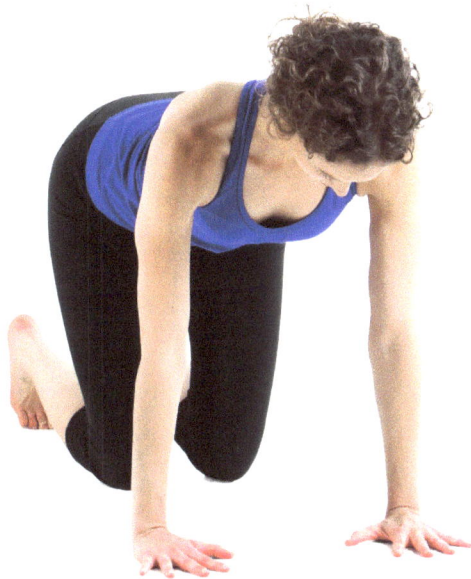

2.1

Sit on your knees next to a wall with your body facing away from the wall.

Place your palms on the floor and slowly walk your feet up the wall until your torso and legs are at a 90 degree angle.

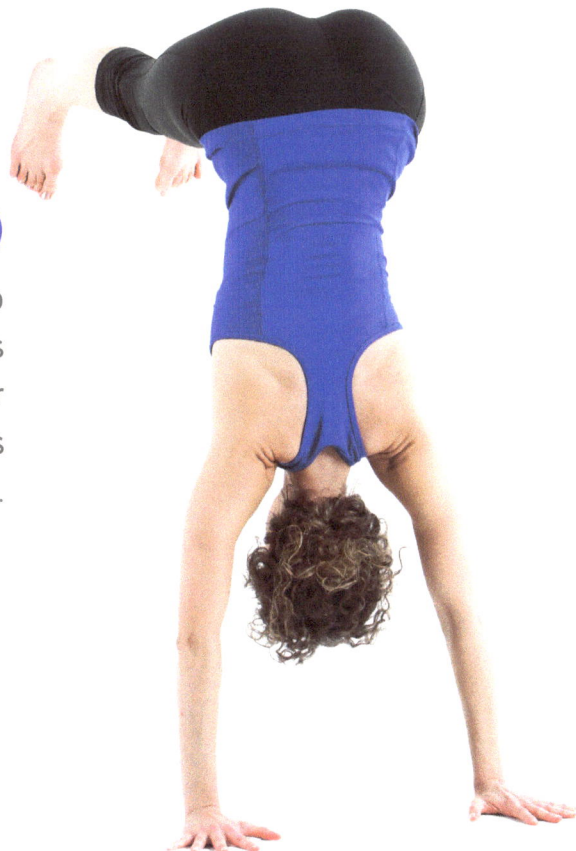

2.2

Press your feet into the wall to help hold the position. Tense both arms and shoulders and your upper back and stomach muscles during the exhalation.

A

Lie down on your back with your legs straight in front of you. Place your arms at your sides with your palms on the floor.

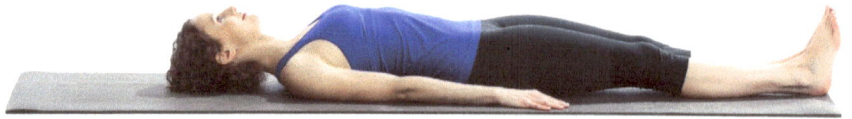

46

B

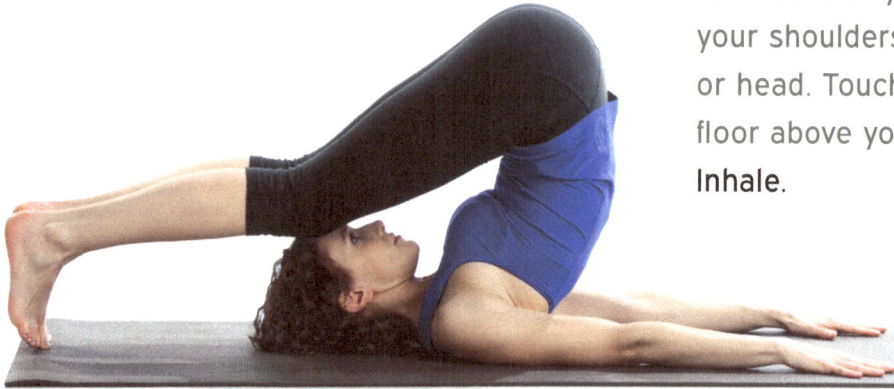

Press your hands into the floor and bring your legs above your head so that your weight is on your shoulders, not your neck or head. Touch your toes on the floor above your head.
Inhale.

C

Exhale as you straighten your legs and press your feet farther behind you for a hamstring and calf stretch.

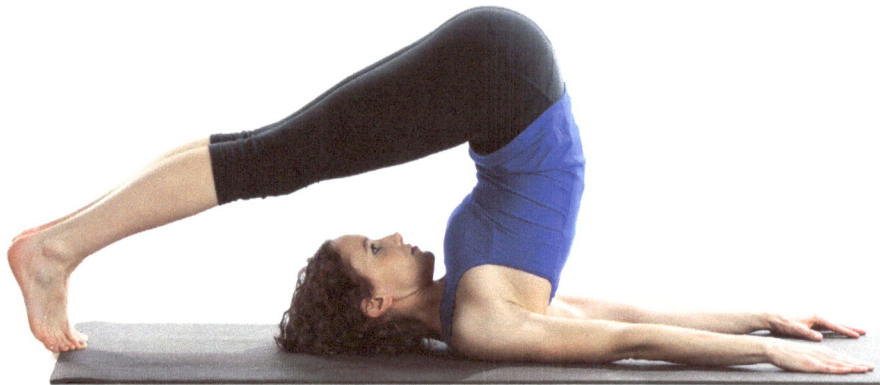

Hold position **C** on each inhalation and stretch farther on each exhalation.

Variation:

1.1

Press your palms into your thighs to help straighten the knees.

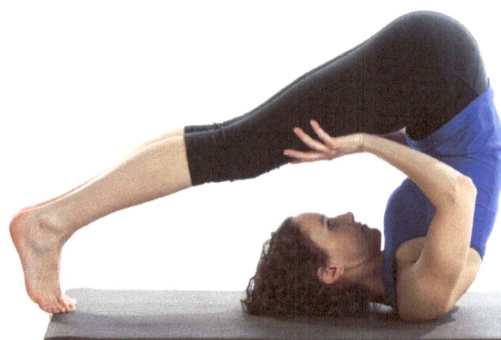

A Sit on your feet with your palms on the floor in front of you. Extend one leg at a time so that you come into a wide legged side split.

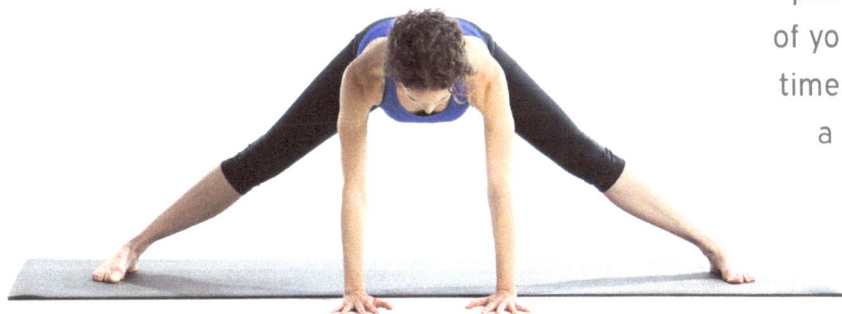

Keep both feet on the floor with your toes pointed forward.

B

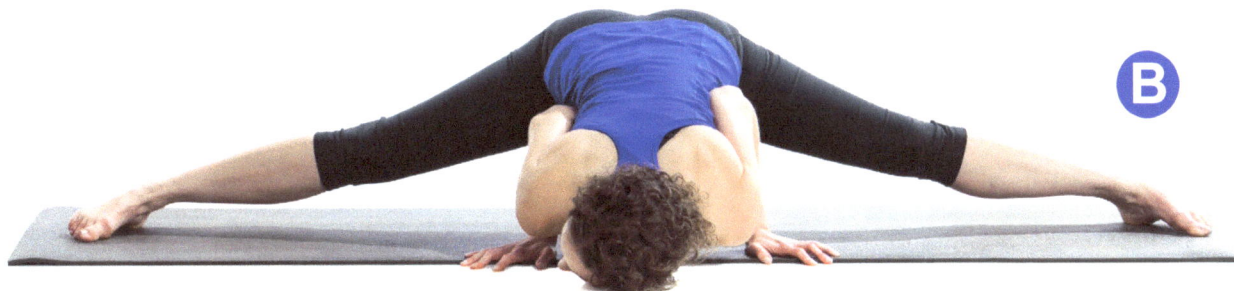

Slide out into the side splits as far as you can and eventually drop your chest to the floor.

Inhale.

C

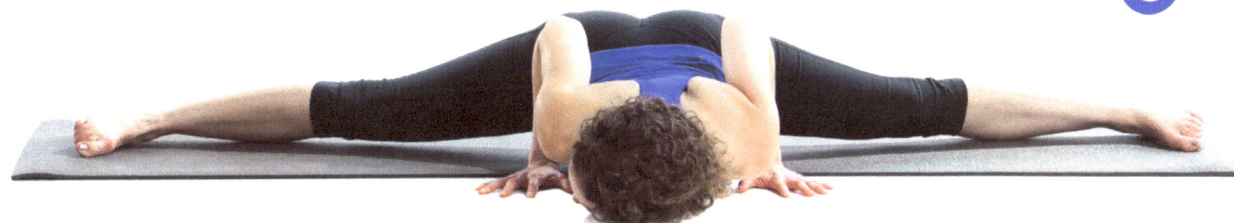

Exhale as you tense your inner thighs and slide farther out into the splits for an inner thigh stretch.

If you cannot isolate the inner thigh, tense your entire thigh and your inner thigh muscles will engage.

Hold position **C** on each inhalation and tense harder and stretch farther on each exhalation.

Variation:

1.1

Lie down on your back at a wall and spread your legs to a side splits on the wall. Tense your inner thighs and use your hands to push your legs farther apart on each exhalation.

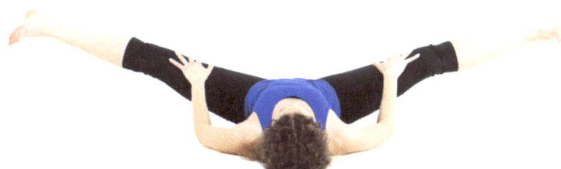

73

A

Kneel down and extend your left leg in front of you.

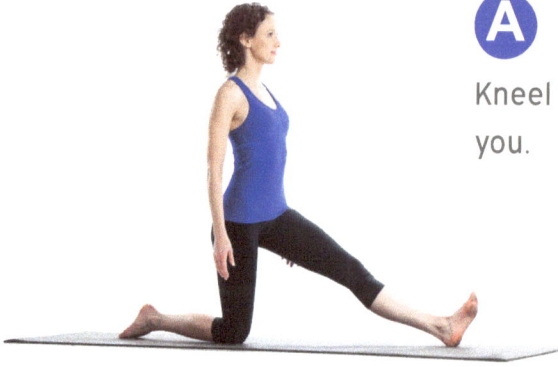

B

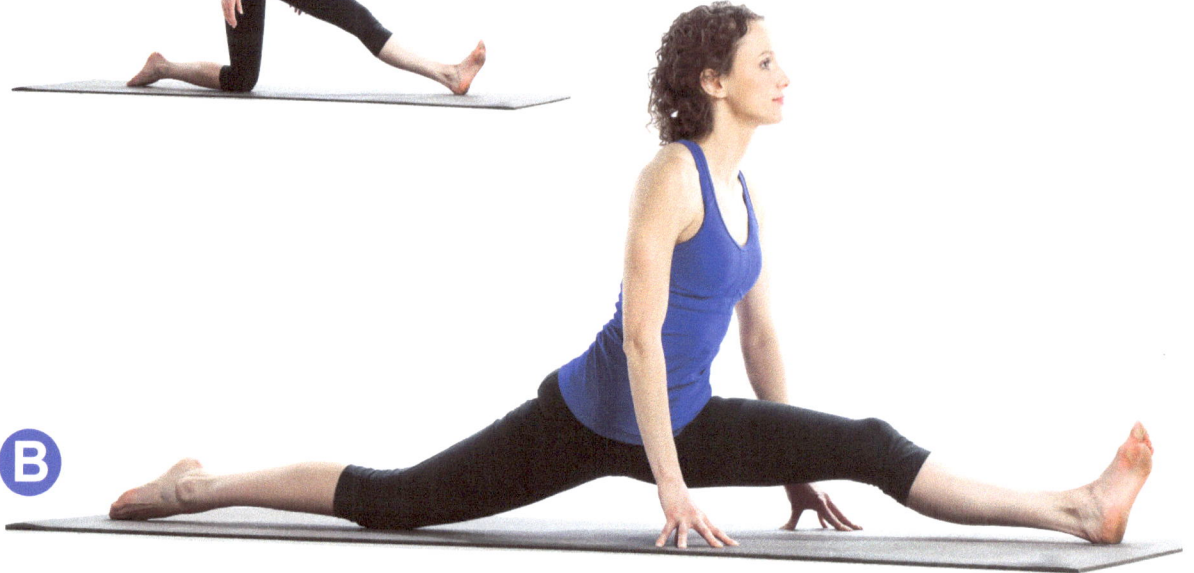

Slide your left foot forward and your right foot back so that you drop down to front splits. Keep the top of the right foot on the floor so that your hips stay in line.

If needed, use your hands for balance on either side of your hips. Keep your spine straight. **Inhale**.

C

Exhale as you tense your left hamstring and your right upper thigh and slide farther out into the front splits for a hamstring and thigh stretch.

If you cannot isolate the hamstring, tense your entire thigh and your hamstring will engage.

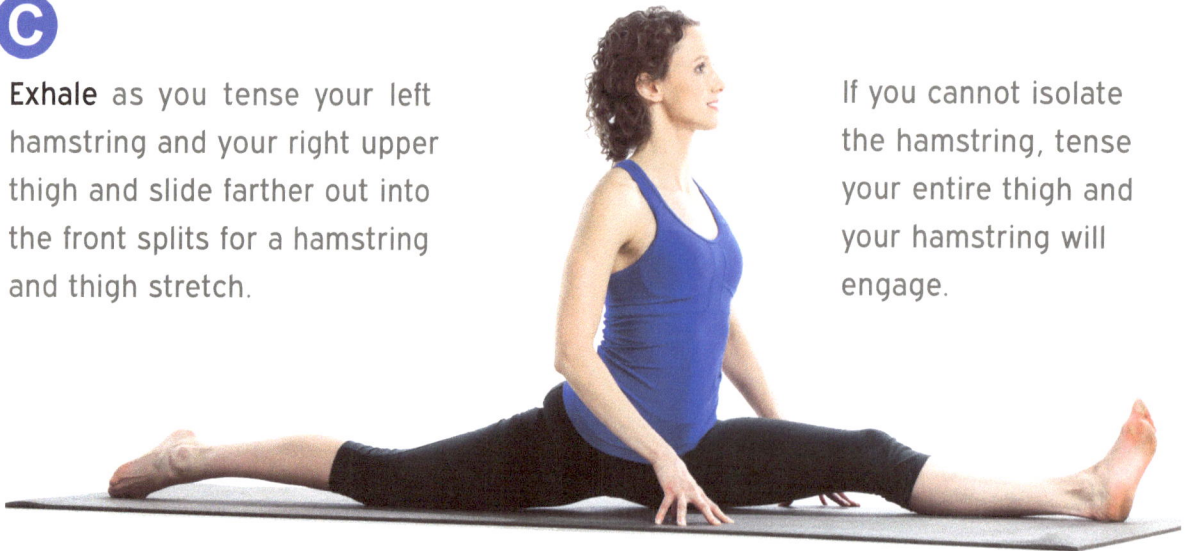

Hold position **C** on each inhalation and tense harder and stretch farther on each exhalation. Repeat on the opposite side for the same number of repetitions.

Variations:

All of the variations here work different aspects of the exercise, so I recommend practicing all the variations regularly.

1.1

Keep the right knee bent and bend over the left hamstring with a straight spine. Tense your left hamstring.

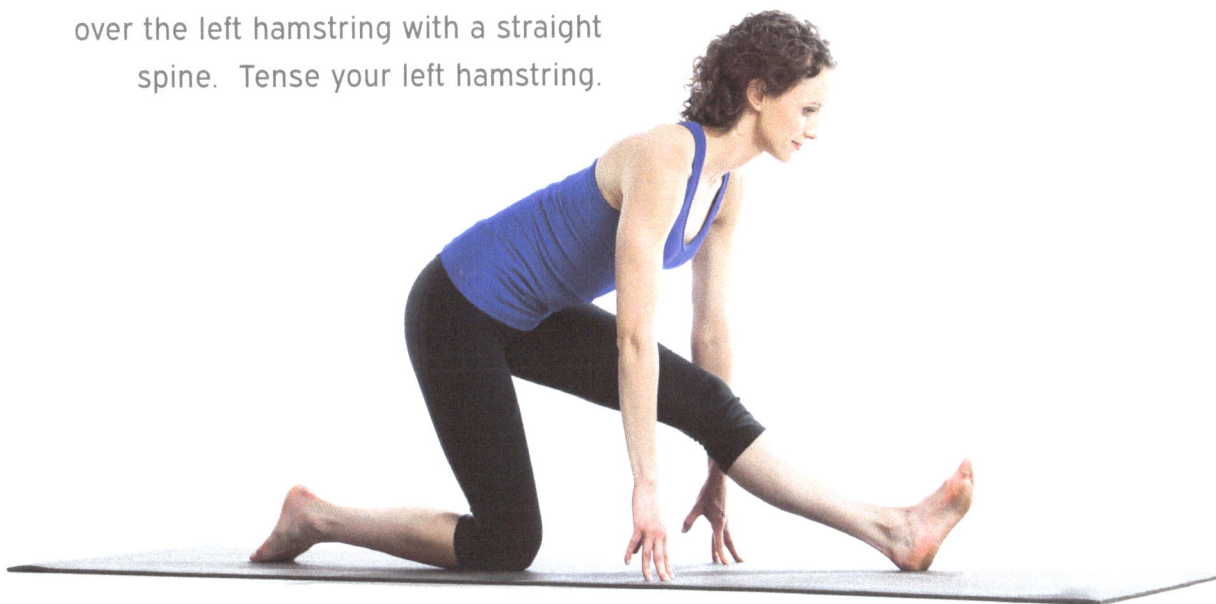

2.1

Bend your left knee and press your weight forward over left foot.

Drop your right hip and thigh towards the floor and lean your chest up and back to put your weight into the right leg.

Tense your right upper thigh.

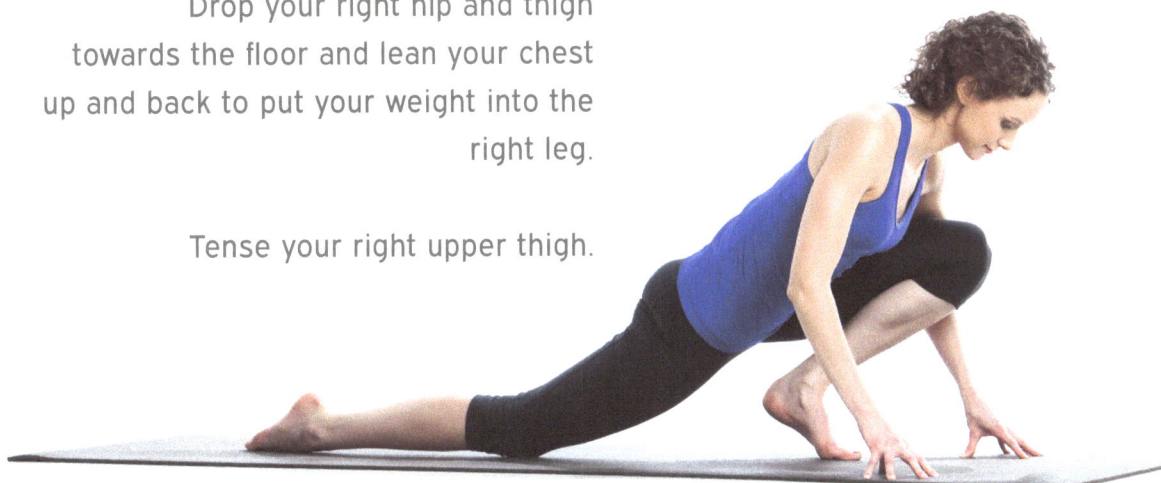

A

Sit on your feet with your knees spread apart. Press your right elbow into the middle of your stomach and place your right palm on the floor in between your legs so that your fingertips point towards your feet.

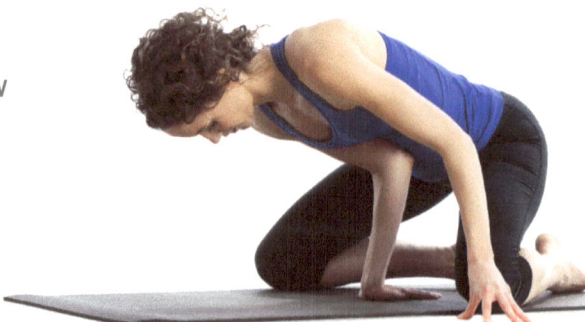

Place your left hand out to the side for balance. **Inhale**.

B

Exhale as you push your weight forward and extend your legs out behind you. Tense your glutes and hamstrings.

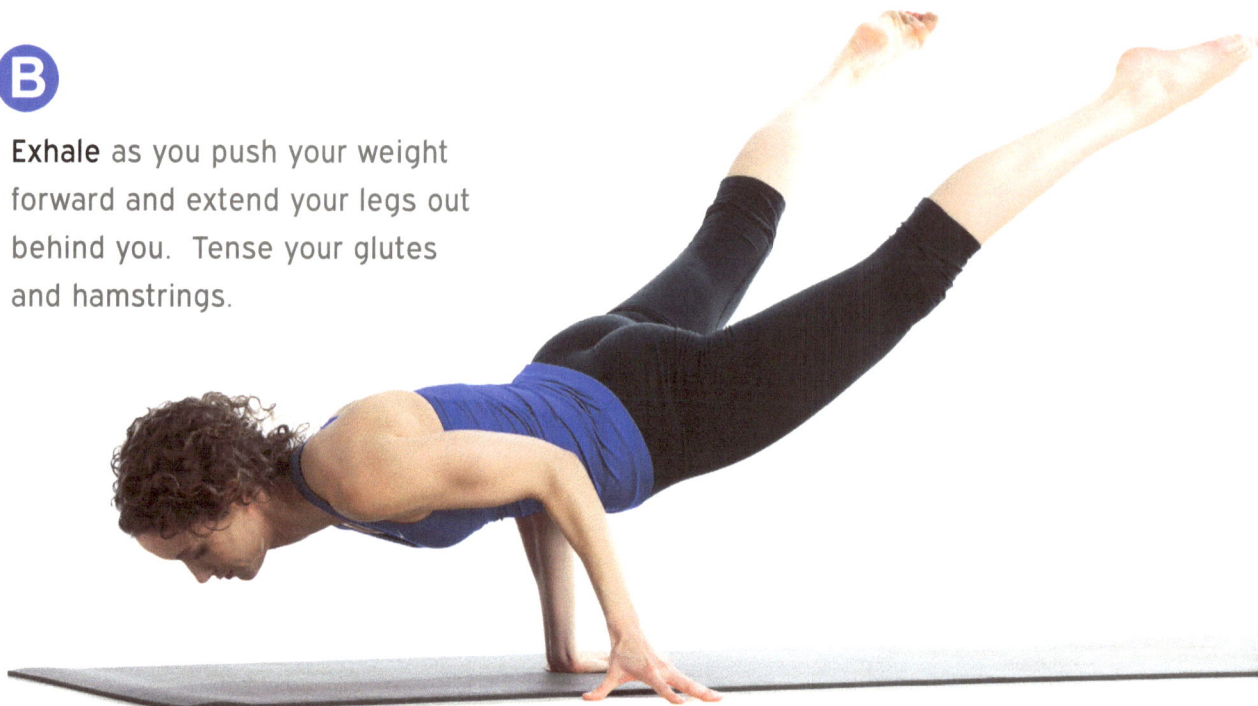

C

Once you achieve balance, lift your left hand off the floor.

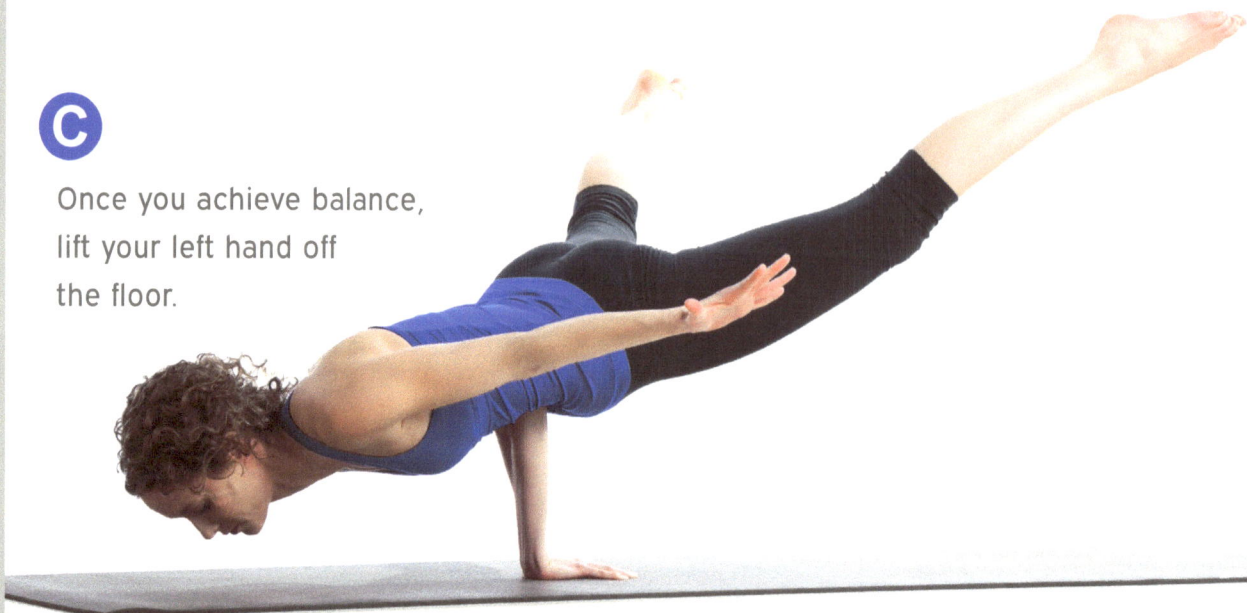

Hold position ⒞ on each inhalation and tense harder on the exhalation. Repeat on the opposite side for the same number of repetitions.

Variation:

I strongly advise not attempting #49 until you have built up wrist strength from regularly practicing many of these exercises such as #1, #2, #25, and any of the arm balance or pushup exercises.

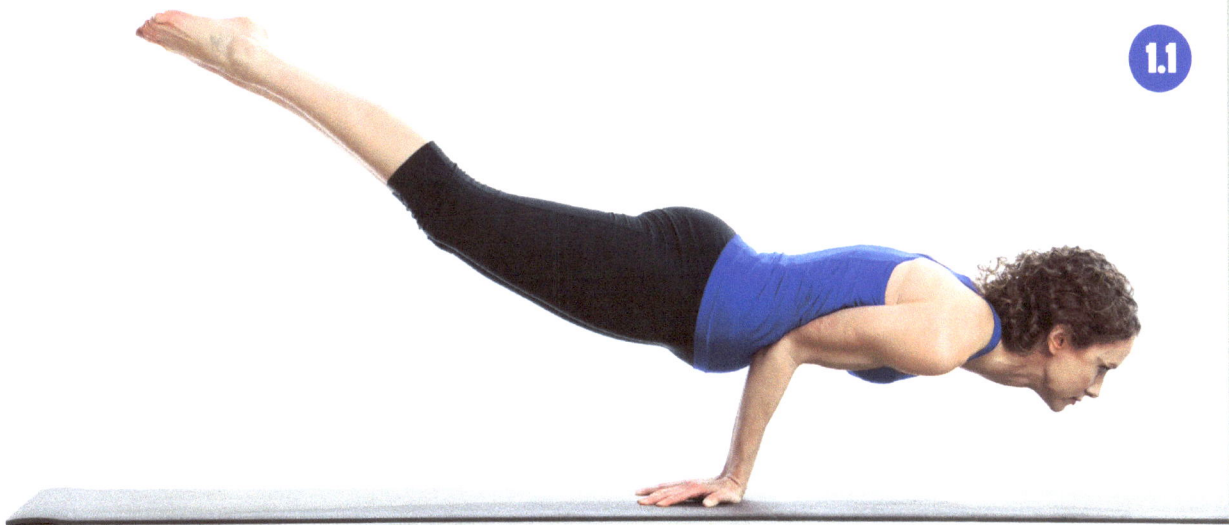

1.1

The 49 I Chin Ching Exercises

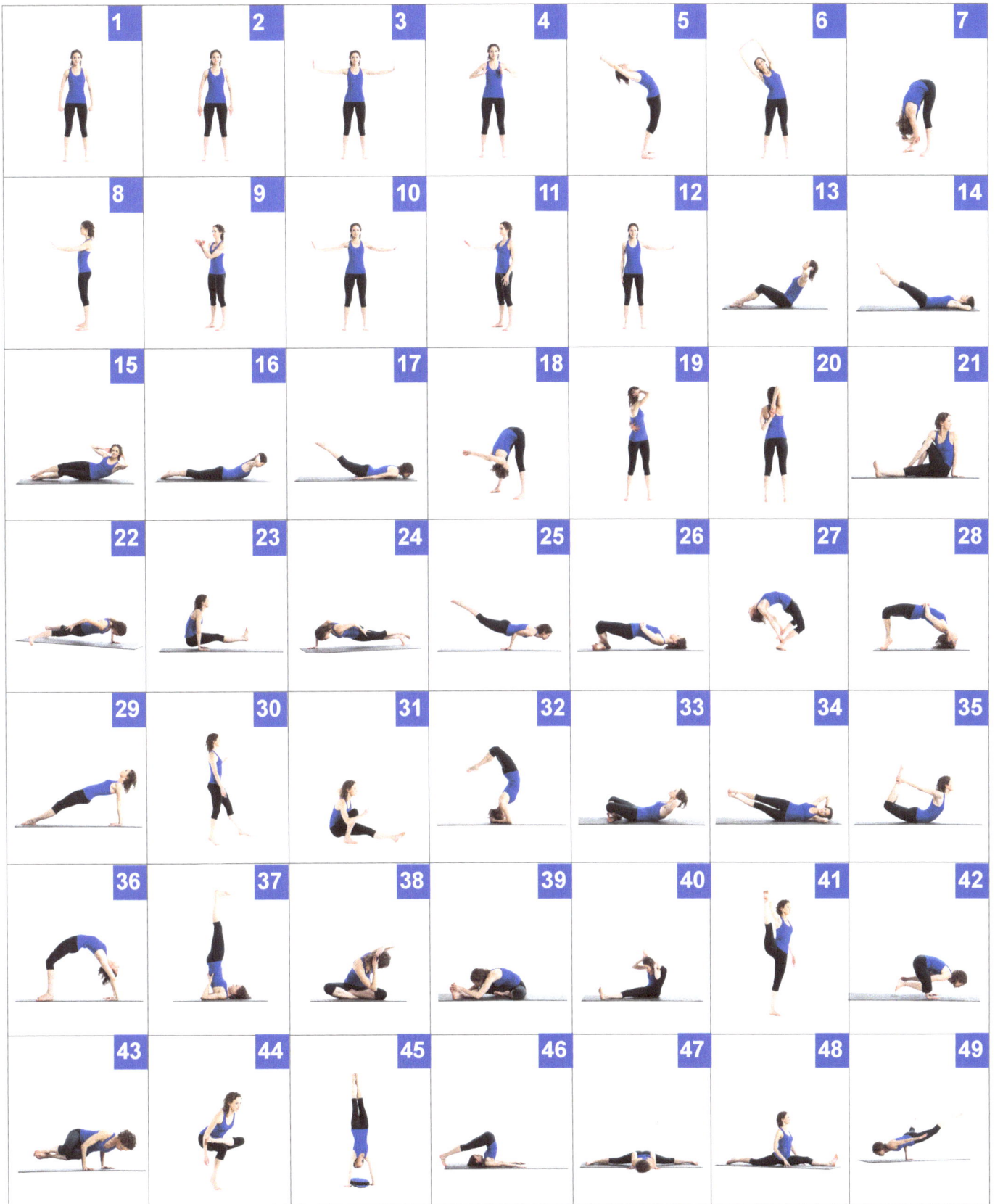

www.ingramcontent.com/pod-product-compliance
Lightning Source LLC
Chambersburg PA
CBHW060805270326
41927CB00002B/61